TOXIC HUMAN FOOD:

Discover How to Reevaluate Your
Dietary Choices and Food Lifestyle

By

Dr. Jerry Forrest

Table of content

INTRODUCTION

Intoxication from food is not known to occur very often. Everyone is aware that particular foods are sometimes blamed for more or less severe "attacks of indigestion" or other physiological changes that have occurred after intake, although the proof in many instances is flimsy at best. The term "ptomain poisoning," which provides a handy haven from etiological ambiguity, has undoubtedly been used to diagnose a wide range of different illnesses, from appendicitis and gallstone pain to simple abdominal distention brought on by careless overeating.

However, it is conceivable that intestinal and other conditions linked to certain foods occur considerably more often than is recognized. There aren't many people who haven't had somewhat uncomfortable gastrointestinal problems that they might easily blame on a recent meal. Identifying the problematic meal with a considerable amount of confidence is often achievable. The vast majority of these assaults are minor in nature, are swiftly treated, and are never reported outside of the close family. Knowledge of the incident only spreads more broadly when the assault is more severe than usual or when a significant number of people are impacted at once. Only a tiny percentage of toxic food cases are documented in medical publications, and only a much smaller percentage of cases are reported to the general press. In fact, only a few are ever fully researched in terms of their genesis.

Even though most cases of toxic food are mild and seem to be transient, this does not mean that they should be dismissed or given little consideration from the perspective of public health. By these assaults, many of which are real illnesses, as we will see, the human body is always somewhat weakened, and as is known to happen with many infectious disorders, some lasting damaging impressions may be left on the body of the sick person.

Acute poisoning, which only lasts a brief period in even the mildest instances, has the potential to start or speed up degenerative changes in the kidneys or blood vessels under certain circumstances.

These alterations may be the result of those sneaky types of toxic food brought on by the repeated consumption of minute amounts of mineral or organic poisons, each of which may not significantly alter physiological function but whose cumulative impact may be harmful. The severity, causes, and methods of preventing toxic food have become urgent research topics given the dire scenario indicated by the rise in degenerative illnesses impacting early middle age in the United States.

CHAPTER ONE

HOW COMMON IS TOXIC FOOD?

Public health authorities often lack information about the prevalence of instances of toxic food, "ptomain poisoning," and similar conditions since they are not required by law to be recorded.

A VARIETY OF TOXIC FOODS

Toxic food cases can be divided into two categories:

1. Those caused by a harmful ingredient in the food itself; and
2. Those caused by a peculiar condition of the person consuming the food, due to which essentially healthy food substances can cause physiological disturbance in some people.

The second category consists of people who are ostensibly normal in other ways but who are more or less negatively impacted by a specific dietary component, such as eggs or milk, which are freely consumed by everyone who is normal. This is the alleged food allergy or sensitivity.

The composition, contents, or contamination of the food itself is what causes toxic food, as it is more commonly recognized. Any of those instances when certain harmful compounds are intentionally introduced to food are beyond the purview of this book. The term "toxic food" is used here to refer to cases of infection brought on by ingesting bacteria and other parasites that infest or contaminate certain foods, as well as the infrequent cases of poisoning from organic poisons present in normal animal or plant tissues and the more or less harmful effects that follow consumption of food into which formed mineral or organic poisons have been introduced accidentally or with the intention of improving appearances or maintaining quality. Little is known regarding the relative frequency of occurrence of these many reasons or the degree to which they are individually and jointly effective, as was previously said.

THE FOOD ITEMS MOST OFTEN ASSOCIATED WITH TOXIC FOOD

In addition to unquestionably deadly plants or animals, several commonplace foods have regularly been linked to more severe outbreaks of toxic food. In broad discussions of this topic, the phrase "meat poisoning" is used approximately as often as "toxic food" due to the prevalence of meat in particular. There is no doubt that the consumption of meat or meat products has been correctly blamed for the vast majority of the best-studied and most severe cases of toxic food. Other animal products, particularly milk and its derivatives, such as cheese and ice cream, have also been blamed for significant and widespread epidemics.

The regularity with which outbreaks of toxic food have been linked to the consumption of raw or improperly prepared food may be considered the most important characteristic of these incidents. The next chapters will address the most likely explanation of this information. A disproportionately high number of incidents of toxic food have been linked to the consumption of raw sausage and uncooked milk, either on their own or in combination with other foods.

Numerous types of canned products have also been frequently accused of having harmful consequences, although the supporting data is not always strong. It is still far from clear how dangerous this source really is. The National Canners Association includes a short summary of "libels on the industry"—cases in which different types of canned goods were blamed for illnesses—in the secretary's annual report. The 1916 report includes 51 incidents of this kind, none of which the Association's investigator found to be supported by solid evidence. It would seem beneficial to do an even more thorough examination into all of these incidents, not in an effort to prove or disprove the innocence of any one product, but rather just to gather all the information and record it.

CHAPTER TWO

AWARENESS OF PROTEIN FOODS

When a tiny amount of egg white or another seemingly safe protein substance is injected under the skin of a guinea pig for the first time, there are no obvious negative effects; however, if the same substance is injected again after an interval of about ten days, the animal will die suddenly and exhibit violent poisoning symptoms. There is no denying that the condition known as protein sensitization or anaphylaxis is rather prevalent, regardless of the physiological reason for the dramatic shift that thus arises from the absorption of foreign proteins into the body. The first discovery of protein sensitization was made via the examination of therapeutic sera, and it has since been shown to have unanticipatedly broad implications.

It is now understood that the reaction to tuberculin and similar side effects of bacterial infection are likely to be explained on the principle of anaphylactic change, in addition to the rash and other symptoms that can occasionally follow the administration of horse serum containing diphtheria antitoxin. Hay fever, which is caused by a person's sensitivity to a specific plant's pollen and is often accompanied by asthma and other anaphylactic symptoms, is another example of a typical case of anaphylaxis.

Infrequent occurrences of sensitivity to certain food ingredients are among the responses often categorized as anaphylaxis. It is a well-known truth that certain foods that most people can consume without consequence are more or less profoundly harmful for others. Strawberries, a few other fruits, and a few types of shellfish are some of the foods that are most often mentioned. It is also highlighted that using eggs and cow's milk might cause unpleasant reactions. The intensity of the episodes might range from a mild rash to severe circulatory, neurological, and gastrointestinal disorders.

Has presented a very typical situation with a kid who is 21 months old, otherwise healthy, but has mild eczema. When the youngster was a little over a year old, egg white was given to it; shortly thereafter, nausea and vomiting set in. A further egg-white feeding took place around eight months later and was immediately followed by sneezing and every sign of severe coryza. The majority of the body had extensive urticaria, and the eyes swelled up. There was no obvious prostration, and the temperature stayed normal. Although the signs and symptoms of such episodes vary greatly from person to person, they often involve significant urticaria coupled with nausea, vomiting, and diarrhea. The speed at which the symptoms start to manifest after eating is really distinctive.

Also, the case of an eight-year-old child who had a clearly visible sensitivity to oatmeal, eggs, and almonds. In this case, experiments revealed that only the proteins in these various meals could cause a response, whereas extracts and preparations devoid of protein were completely inactive. It was also shown that guinea pigs may be passively sensitized against the drugs in issue by injecting the patient's blood serum, proving the condition to be one of true anaphylaxis.

Infants may show idiosyncrasies to cow's milk, which is an allergic occurrence. In these situations, switching to goat's milk from cow's milk has shown positive outcomes.

An approach to therapy based on animal experiments has been recommended in really problematic instances of protein idiosyncrasy. This involves producing "anti-anaphylaxis" by the systematic administration of small quantities of the relevant protein ingredient. The instance of a kid who had a constitutional response after receiving one teaspoonful of a solution made up of one pint of water and one drop of egg white but who was perfectly able to take the same quantity of albumen diluted with one quart of water The infant was progressively given increasing volumes of stronger solutions, starting with the dilution that didn't cause a response. The dose was always one teaspoon, given three times daily. As a consequence, the youngster became so desensitized over the course of around three months that one dram of pure egg white may now be consumed guilt-free.

The quantity of the particular protein required in some of these situations to trigger the reaction is quite tiny. A doctor describes a patient who "could not tolerate the slightest quantity of egg in any form. He had severe nausea and violent vomiting if a spoon was used to whip eggs and then mix his coffee.

It is a known fact that many "asthma" cases rely on certain meals. Sensitization to particular meals is also linked to a variety of skin rashes and eruptions.

Each specific food (such as cereals or tomatoes) causes a consistent and unique set of symptoms.

This kind of toxic food may cause some skin conditions that are perhaps identifiable. By using cutaneous and intracutaneous testing, it was shown that just one of the forty-three individuals without eczema exhibited any signs of vulnerability to proteins, but twenty-two of the twenty-seven patients with eczema did.

CHAPTER THREE

POISONOUS ANIMALS AND PLANT LIFE

Normal plant and animal tissues commonly mistaken for healthy meals include chemicals that are harmful to humans.

HARMFUL PLANT LIFE

Sometimes poisonous plants make a prominent appearance in human affairs.

Every student of ancient history is familiar with the tale of Socrates who "drank the hemlock," and they are also aware of the cunning imperial killers who would often use deadly mushrooms in place of edible ones in the meals they cooked for visitors who were unpopular. Today, poisoning from ingesting toxic plants mostly results from an accident, and it primarily affects children and the uninformed.

Heller's "Catalogue of North American Plants" lists 16,673 leaf-bearing plants, and it has been claimed that roughly 500 of them are dangerous in some form.

Some of these are relatively uncommon or unlikely to be consumed by humans or animals for other reasons; others only have a poison in a specific area or are only toxic during certain times of the year; still others only have a poison that is dangerous when it comes into contact with the skin, is injected beneath the skin, or is injected into the bloodstream. Individual vulnerability to some of these plant toxins varies greatly. Even when handled carelessly, a common plant known as "poison ivy" is not toxic to many humans and is safe for most domestic animals to consume.

The real number of hazardous plants that people are actually likely to unintentionally ingest is not that high. The United States is home to over thirty significant poisonous plants, some of which are only toxic to domestic animals.

Many of the recorded incidents of human poisoning fall into the category of very unusual mishaps and have no bearing on the current issue. These include accidentally using daffodil bulbs as food, mistaking young broad-leaf laurel (Kalmia latifolia) shoots for wintergreen, mistaking the leaves of the American false hellebore (**Veratrum viride**) for those of the marsh marigold, and mistaking the fruit pulp of the Kentucky coffee tree (**Gymnocladus dioica**) for that of the honey locust. The use of the spindle-shaped roots of the deadly water hemlock (**Cicuta maculata**), which is related to the more well-known but no more lethal poison hemlock, is one of the most severe cases of poisoning of this kind. Children confuse these subterranean plant parts, which are sometimes visible due to freezing or washing, for food roots like horseradish, artichokes, and parsnips. There are likely more cases of water hemlock poisoning than are documented.

There were eight instances and two fatalities from this cause in the state of New Jersey alone in one year.

The epidemic in Hamburg and around 30 other German towns brought on by the use of a deadly vegetable fat in the preparation of a commercial butter replacement is an example of toxic food to be included under this heading. The makers have added a variety of plant oils to the margarine formulation in an effort to keep costs as low as feasible. The poisoning in the Hamburg incident, which resulted in over 200 instances of sickness, was reportedly brought on by the replacement of so-called ***maratti oil***, which is produced from a tropical plant (**Hydrocarpus**).

According to a claim that it is the same as ***cardamom oil***, this fat is harmful in the quantities used in margarine, as shown by an animal experiment. If necessary measures aren't taken while testing novel fats and other untested compounds intended for use in the manufacturing of food items, rising economic demand for inexpensive meals might result in the recurrence of such incidents.

The New York City Health Department's investigators have discovered that several instances of purported "ptomain poisoning" were really caused by "sour-grass soup." This soup is made from the oxalic acid-rich leaves of a sorrel species. One restaurant's soup was discovered to have up to 10 grains of oxalic acid per pint!

Hazardous mushrooms are by far the best-known example of the kind of poisoning that happens when edible and hazardous items are mistakenly consumed. There is reason to believe that the frequency of mushroom (or "toadstool") intoxication in the United States has increased recently. This may be due in part to the fact that more people are eating mushrooms as food on a regular basis, which increases the risk of error, as well as the rise in immigration from Southern European communities that regularly consume mushrooms. Numerous cases of immigrants mistaking toxic types in this nation for edible ones they were used to in their native countries have come to light. Twenty-two people in the region of New York City died from mushroom poisoning over the course of 10 days as a result of heavy rains. In this nation, the "fly Amanita" (*AA manita muscaria*) is reportedly often confused with the European form of "royal Amanita" (*AA. caesaria*). The Count de Vecchi's apparent cause of death in Washington, D.C., in 1897 seems to have been due to such an error.

The Count, an attaché of the Italian legation and a well-bred man close to sixty years old who was regarded as somewhat of an authority on mycology, bought a number of fungi near one of the marketplaces in Washington that he identified as edible mushrooms. The plants were gathered in Virginia, seven miles from Washington, D.C. The count and his doctor, a dear personal friend, had breakfast together the next Sunday and remarked on the mushrooms' acceptable, even delectable taste. After breakfast was over at half past eight, the count began to experience signs of a severe sickness within fifteen minutes. The beginning was so sudden that by nine in the morning, he was discovered face down on his bed, overcome with dread. He quickly started losing consciousness, experienced trismus, became blind, and had trouble eating. Then terrible convulsions took over, which were so strong that they broke the bed on which he was lying. The count died the day after the accident, never regaining consciousness despite intensive care and the use of morphine and atropine. When the count's doctor arrived back at his office, he too was attacked, with dizziness and eye symptoms alerting him to the severity of the problem. His coworkers immediately started energetic treatment with apomorphine and atropine, and for the next five hours he was in a coma with sporadic episodes of awareness. The severe symptoms were reduced, and at seven o'clock in the evening, recovery began. His recovery went without a hitch; he was fully recovered, and I think he is still alive. The count in this case most likely identified the fungus as Caesaria or Aurantiaca. The species ingested must have been a Muscaria species based on the symptoms and termination.

An alkaloidal compound found in A. muscaria has been given the name muscarin and the precise chemical formula **$C_5H_{15}NO_3$**, and it has a distinctive impact on the nerve centers. **Atropin** is a medication that has been used successfully in instances of muscarinic poisoning since it is a more-or-less perfect physiological antidote for the toxin. According to legend, Caucasian peasants had a custom of making a drink called "Amanita" from flies, which they employed to induce drunken orgies. It is said that numerous deaths result from consuming this beverage in excess.

The majority of instances of mushroom poisoning are presumably caused by the dangerous _Amanita_ or death cup (A. phalloides). Ford calculates that only one species alone is responsible for twelve to fifteen fatalities every year in this nation. Usually, people who have collected and eaten whatever they happened to find in the woods consume this fungus out of simple ignorance. A family's demise might result from a handful of these lethal mushrooms mixed with edible types.

Description of the signs of A. phalloides poisoning:

After eating the mushrooms, there is a six- to fifteen-hour window during which the victims do not exhibit any signs of poisoning. This is comparable to the incubation time for other intoxications or diseases. The first indication of difficulty is abrupt, severe abdominal discomfort that is localized, followed by vomiting, thirst, and cholera-like diarrhea with mucus and bloody stools. By no means is the latter symptom continuous. The agony persists in paroxysms that are often so intense that they result in the unusual Hippocratic facies, or "la face vultueuse" in French, and even when it sometimes becomes better in nature, it typically returns with increased intensity.

The patients swiftly lose muscle and strength, and their skin begins to take on an odd yellow tone. Children and adults go into a deep coma after three to four days and between six and eight days, respectively. Death swiftly puts an end to this terrifying and pointless tragedy. Rarely, if ever, do convulsions happen, and when they do, they suggest a combination of intoxication from eating phalloides and Amanita muscaria specimens, in my opinion. Although recovery is not always possible when small amounts of the fungus are consumed, especially if the stomach is very promptly emptied, either naturally or artificially, mortality rates for those poisoned by the "deadly Amanita" range from 60 to 100% in various accidents.

Other closely related Amanita species, such as A. verna, the "destroying angel," which is possibly a smaller version of A. phalloides, have a toxic effect that is comparable to that of A. phalloides.

The nature of the toxin was first thoroughly examined. Extract from amanita has the ability to remove or dissolve the pigment from red blood cells. Even at a dilution of 1:125,000, its hemolytic effect is so potent that it affects the red cells of oxblood. Ford has recently shown that this species of Amanita also contains a compound that is far more toxic than the hemolytic substance, and he draws the conclusion that this substance, known as the "Amanita toxin," is principally responsible for the fungus' harmful effects. The juice of the cooked "Amanita" has no hemolytic properties, but it is dangerous to animals in tiny amounts, which is consistent with the finding that these mushrooms are still very poisonous to humans even after being cooked. The real "Amanita" toxin causes extensive fatty degeneration in the liver, kidneys, and heart muscle.

The most intriguing functional alterations were seen in the kidney rather than the liver. These writers come to the conclusion that, rather than being brought on by some strange "neurotoxin," the neurological and mental symptoms are likely uremic in nature. There are no known effective therapy options. Although a hemolysin antibody has been created, very little antitoxin for the other toxic chemical seems to be developing. Only a tiny portion of attempts to immunize small animals with amanite toxin are successful.

TOXIC ANIMAL

Although many animal muscles and internal organs are unpleasant to consume, there don't appear to be any that are harsh or have a poor taste, as they are edible. Eating ordinary animal tissues may be hazardous in a number of situations.

The majority of meat-related outbreaks, the existence of dangerous microorganisms, or exposure to toxins produced after the animal's death are what cause sea toxic food. because it has been shown to be very accurate in a number of poisoning incidents.

Mollusks that were implicated originated from water that had been polluted by human feces in the great majority, if not all, of the cases where oysters and other shellfish were blamed.

However, certain animals, notably some fish, have clearly poisonous, active, and healthy organs. the Tetrodontidae family of puffers.

The balloon-fish and globe-fish families include a number of poisonous species. Among them is the well-known Japanese film "Fugu," which features hundreds of deaths. It has been successfully used to stop suicide several times.

Fish species seem to be more diverse in tropical waters than in other kinds of waterways. However, it could be because fish is consumed more often and carelessly as food in areas like Japan and the South Sea Islands. It is well known that certain fish in frigid waters are toxic. The meat of the Greenland shark contains dangerous chemicals characteristics of dogs that make people think of inebriated animals.

There is a lot of confusion about the conditions under which fish poisoning may manifest itself in a variety of ways. One kind claims that reproductive tissues are accessible and connected to the spawning season, with a possible connection to poison. According to reports, European barbel roe often causes poisoning, but usually not serious poisoning. When it comes time for spawning, the flesh or roe of sturgeon, pike, and other fish is also said to be hazardous. It's said that certain fish are poisonous only after they've consumed certain marine plants.

There isn't much information for sure on the chemicals at issue. Nature is definitely not uniform. Seizures, paralysis, and other cholera-like symptoms are brought on by the Fugu toxin. It is not destroyed by boiling.

Greenland shark meat is reported to have the following effects on dogs:

Reports state that dogs are given an ever-increasing

Immunity is developed in certain areas of the poisonous shark's flesh.

Various symptoms of sea toxic food have been reported in the past.

CHAPTER FOUR

ADDED POISONS TO FOOD, EITHER ORGANIC OR MINERAL

Known mineral or organic toxins are referred to as "***chemical poisons***". This find their way into food, either accidentally or intentionally, during the production, preparation, or addition of processes with the aim of improving the meal's appearance or storage capacity.

ARSENIC

Sometimes stupidity or carelessness have resulted in the addition of a poison with the potency of arsenic. Arsenic was discovered by English people authorities to be commonly found in materials that have been treated with sulfuric acid during the preparation process, as well as in materials that have been roasted or dried utilizing gases generated by coal combustion. The same source is used in both scenarios: iron pyrites, which are virtually always arsenic either a part of coal or a method for producing sulfuric acid.

There was a well-known "peripheral neuritis" epidemic in the English Midlands.

Arsenic in potentially dangerous amounts was first identified in 1900.

BEER

About 6,000 individuals were affected by this outbreak, and about 70 people died. The beer that the supposed bar is serving.

Brewing sugars have been used to create all of the breweries. These sugars came from a single source and were found to be arsenic-impregnated because sulfuric acid was utilized in their production. Arsenic concentrations in certain acid samples reached as high as 2.6% during processing.

Strong criticism is leveled at the inclusion of or adulteration with glucose in products like jams, syrups, candies, and the like, not only beer.

Unless it is known that the glucose produced from the contaminated arsenic was made using sulfuric acid. In reality, only sulfuric acid-based meals that employ acid that is devoid of arsenic are allowed for consumption.

ANTIMONY

Antimony, which is noticeable in amounts when cooking a range of foods, is present in the poorer-grade enameled cookware types that are now used in this country. The rubber nipples used to give bottles to babies may also contain antimony, despite the risk.

Although the consequences of repeated, very low concentrations of antimony are recognized, there is little information on these effects. Chronic antimony poisoning has very rarely been documented.

LEAD

Due to the well-known poisonousness of lead and its derivatives, lead salts are purposefully added to dietary products, even in small amounts. True, lead chromate sometimes serves as a yellow tinting agent.

Colorize the sugar used to decorate sweets. food products presented in foods that don't have foil, such as soft cheese and chocolate, however, lead may be found in the contents of preserve jars with metal lids and in "soft drinks" marketed in bottles with patented metal stoppers. Occasional lead in small doses may be eaten without any ill effects.

Physiological relevance since lead is a poison that accumulates over time. Even very small amounts ingested repeatedly constitute a danger. It is well known that regular use of lead may result in serious lead poisoning.

Contains acidic beverages in bottles with a lead cork. Cooking utensils made of glazed and earthenware have been the subject of studies to determine the danger of lead poisoning ingestion, and those studies have shown harm.

This source doesn't seem likely. This country's typical enameled ceramics are lead-free.

A complaint has been raised about the solder-sealed food cans' potential for contamination. These arguments are weaker than others. Due to design changes made to the container, any solder contact with food is now greatly and drastically minimized, if not altogether eradicated.

Using lead is not advised since many natural streams are hostile to it.

Lead poisoning outbreaks have often happened as a consequence of the use of lead service pipes in wells, cisterns, and the public water supply. It is generally agreed that lead pipes should not be used to draw water intended for human consumption.

People have a special susceptibility to ingesting lead via their stomachs. Employing lead salts while working in the painting industry and other contact-based occupations. It has been shown that eating food exposes one to a significant quantity of lead, which, when consumed over an extended period of time, causes lead poisoning. This could make it more likely that lead will contaminate food be considerably decreased by washing hands thoroughly with hot water and soap. Drink water before a meal.

TIN

In a description of the widespread usage of tinned foods, much attention has been paid to the risk of tin poisoning. It's been demonstrated.

Tin damages acidic fruits and berries chemically; however, other plants may only produce a minor acid reaction. Greater amounts of tin are present in the solids after draining than in the alcohol.

In an insoluble condition. Based on research , it has long been held that the quantities of tin typically detected in canned goods "are undeserving of serious notice," and this belief has been reflected in the top hygiene textbooks.

Certainly, the massive rise in the consumption of canned goods has not been accompanied by any appreciable quantity of tin poisoning. However, Friedmann attributes a case of canned asparagus poisoning to the tin content, and this conclusion is supported by the negative findings of his bacteriological and serological tests. It seems that soluble tin compounds are present in an extremely high proportion in canned asparagus. There seems to be some support for the hypothesis that certain people are particularly sensitive to trace amounts of tin and that this is the best explanation for the relative rarity of instances like the one reported by Friedmann. Fruits and vegetables that are particularly prone to attacking tin are increasingly being packaged in lacquered or "enamel-lined" cans.

Though protochloride of tin is said to sometimes be added to molasses in order to reduce the color, the intentional addition of tin salts to food components does not seem to be prevalent. The procedure is not ideal for a number of reasons, including the fact that the chlorides are thought to be more hazardous than other tin compounds. Sanitarians believe that chemicals that might irritate human tissues during digestion or excretion shouldn't be used in food.

Even a small amount of each new irritant may add to the stress already placed on organs due to aging or past harsh treatment.

COPPER

Scientific Experts notes that this substance is far less toxic than it was once believed to be, and he considers it likely that the cases of illness attributed to "verdigris poisoning" reported in the older literature actually occurred. Verdigris, or copper acetate, is a substance that is sometimes formed during cooking, especially during the long standing of certain foods in copper vessels.

The technique of using copper sulfate to give several crops, including peas, beans, and asparagus, a green hue is comparatively new, having begun in France about 1850. Since heat partially destroys or changes the natural green of vegetables, restoring the hue has appealed to certain customers' sense of color. It must be acknowledged that there is some health risk associated with this visual delight. According to Long's tests, copper is absorbed and stored in certain organs, and even modest doses taken often may have a negative effect. He comes to the conclusion that using copper salts to color food must be avoided at all costs. The government of the United States currently forbids the interstate commerce of these chemicals as well as the importation of food colored with copper.

DIFFERENT COLORING AGENTS

Copper sulfate is only one of a number of chemical compounds used to change the natural color of a variety of foods. When dark-colored flour is bleached white using nitrogen peroxide, for example, the public's perception may be that a food product's beauty is boosted by special treatment. However, in many situations, the color alteration is based on absurdly unrealistic criteria. If justified at all, the use of toxic aniline dyes for coloring candy every color of the rainbow must be justified on the basis of aesthetics rather than hygienic considerations. Some commonly used coloring agents, such as annatto, which is always used to color butter, are thought to have no negative health effects, while other agents, like copper sulfate, should always be looked at with skepticism. The best-case scenario for food coloring includes waste and maybe major health risks. In general, any alteration of the food's natural hue is based on an absurd custom and should be outlawed for the good of the populace. Natural, unprocessed ingredients are much more attractive as foods than bleached wheat, discolored butter, dyed jelly, and ice cream; in fact, they are basically less desirable. Artificially colored meals would not be very palatable if the public were aware of the whole process of food coloring.

Economically speaking, the activity is completely useless. The additional levy of fifty cents to a dollar per barrel is barely worth the artificial flour whitening using potentially dangerous nitrogen peroxide. The nutritional or digestive characteristics of flour are not improved by such bleaching with a noxious gas, and it may even be dangerously harmful. A program of educational enlightenment that will make natural foods look more appetizing than those offered under deceptive hues seems to be the answer to the issue of food coloring. Custom, on the other hand, presents a significant barrier to change in this industry since it is supported by effective advertising.

PRESERVATIVES FOR FOOD

Keeping food in reserve from a time of abundance to a time of shortage is not only acceptable but also highly recommended. Food has been preserved throughout history by methods including drying, smoking, salting, and, more recently, refrigeration and heat (canning). These later techniques have increasingly begun to influence how civilized cultures eat. All techniques of preservation are based on the elimination of microbes or the restriction of their development by different physical and chemical agents, since microbic activity is what causes food to decay. It has long been accepted to utilize some chemical preservatives, such as saltpeter brines, acid pickles, and strong sugar and salt solutions. The use of chemical preservatives has recently taken on a new dimension as a result of manufacturers' growing propensity to add antiseptic chemicals—which come in a range of forms and have questionable physiological effects—to food goods.

Declaring that no dangerous material should be introduced to food is not as straightforward and simple as it may seem. The quantity and kind of material are both factors in the scientific definition of a poison. Large quantities of common salt are deadly, but as we all know, small amounts are not only safe but also vital for health. Strychnine and quinine, two well-known and very potent protoplasmic poisons, are often supplied in very small quantities for medical reasons without producing any harmful effects.

Smoked meats and fish, which get their preservation properties from the creosote and other compounds that the smoke impregnates them with, demonstrate how difficult the issue of employing food preservatives really is. Although there has been little to no opposition to the use of smoked foods, despite the fact that these ingredients are significantly more dangerous than artificial preservatives like benzoic acid, about which great worry has been raised,

Benzoic acid (also known as benzoate of soda) is used as a food preservative, which highlights several stages of the debate. Benzoate of soda supplied with meals was supposed to cause "a very serious disturbance of the metabolic functions, attended with injury to digestion and health." However, the trials of the Referee Board of

Scientific Experts (1909), which were carried out with at least similar care and diligence, were seen to support the following assertions:

1. Sodium benzoate, when coupled with food in tiny dosages (less than five tenths of a gram per day), has no harmful or hazardous effects and is not harmful to health.

2. It has not been shown that significant dosages of sodium benzoate, up to four grams per day, taken with food, have any negative effects on the general health or behave as a poison in the traditional sense of the word. Certain physiological systems underwent small adjustments in various areas, the precise relevance of which is unknown.

3. It has not been determined that the addition of sodium benzoate, whether in small or large dosages, to food would harm or degrade the meal's quality or nutritional value.

Even more research conducted under the sponsorship of the German government revealed that in order to produce any observable effects in dogs and rabbits, relatively high doses of benzoic acid (equivalent to 60 to 100 grams per day for a man weighing 150 pounds) were required. This result might be seen as a general confirmation of the Referee Board's conclusion that four grams per day is safe.

Probably the strongest argument for the usage of any chemical compound at the moment is given by the facts on the impact of benzoic acids and benzoates when used as food preservatives. Many fruits and berries, particularly cranberries, contain benzoic acid in notable concentrations, and its presence in these unprocessed foods has never been linked to any harmful effects.

In actuality, chemicals found in a variety of common meals are transformed by the body into hippuric acid and ultimately benzoic acid.

We are aware that small amounts of benzoic acid and benzoic acid compounds found in food or produced by the body can be handled and rendered harmless by the human body. We are also aware of how this is done and reasonably certain of which organ is responsible. We also know that the process by which the harmful hippuric acid is transformed into the toxic benzoic acid is very effective and capable of handling rather large amounts of benzoic acid. The typical animal organism is more than capable of carrying out the necessary function in this instance, as well as in a huge number of others. From this perspective, it may be claimed, and it has been argued strongly, that the human body is more than capable of turning harmless levels of benzoic acid or benzoate that are added to some items of our food for preservation into acceptable levels.

This viewpoint, in my opinion, will win out, and the conflict will turn into a debate about how much benzoic acid should be allowed to enter our daily food supply.

However, we should exercise extreme caution before adopting any precise number, especially one that is significant, as the maximum allowable level of added benzoic acid in our meals. The fact that we have a reliable method for changing dangerous benzoic acid into safe hippuric acid suggests that this process is necessary only by virtue of the fact that we have it. It implies that even trace amounts of benzoic acid that we consume in naturally occurring foods or manufacture inside ourselves might be harmful to our health if not for the mechanism that forms hippuric acid, which protects us. Furthermore, just because there is a significant "factor of safety" in relation to the typical benzoic acid concentration of our diet, it does not imply that we may trespass on it without consequence. A few rather brief feeding tests cannot tell us what the outcome of a widespread, ongoing encroachment on it would be. It is well recognized that although certain chemicals may be used in large doses for a month or a year without showing any clearly harmful consequences, continuing to consume the same compounds, even in reduced amounts, can ultimately harm one's health. It may be better to get the ultimate answer to the benzoic acid issue straight from the general public. It would not take more than a decade or two before we should have a well-defined and well-founded public opinion on the subject, at least in the medical profession, if they were to consume benzoic acid as knowingly as they consume, for example, sodic carbonate in soda biscuits or caffeine and theobromine in coffee and tea.

The defense of their safety is much more challenging when compared to other well-known and perhaps toxic food preservatives. *Formaldehyde, salicylic acid, sulfurous acid, and sulfite* are substances that are unquestionably hazardous in relatively tiny concentrations; in animal trials, their harmful effects in minute consecutive dosages are rather pronounced; and their usage in human food items is essentially without rationale. Although they may be somewhat different, borax and boric acid are never found in natural foods, and there is no solid proof that consuming them over an extended period of time in tiny dosages won't have any negative effects. Remember that all of these chemicals' ability to preserve or be antiseptic comes from their toxic impact on bacterial protoplasm. It is reasonable to assume that, in general, bacterial protoplasm is no more easily injured than human protoplasm, which immediately calls into question the propriety of repeatedly exposing human tissues to substances that are likely to cause injury, even if the injury is minor and healing is typically simple. The burden of evidence should always fall squarely on those who support the use of bacterial inhibitors in food meant for human consumption. They must demonstrate that compounds potent enough to prevent the growth of germs are nonetheless unable to significantly affect how human body cells function.

When this point of view is adopted, many home preservatives that have long been accepted as standard practice are also placed under some doubt, in addition to the chemical compounds already described. As far as we are aware, spices like cinnamon, oil of cloves, and the like are just as likely to cause physiological harm when used regularly in tiny doses as some of the "chemical" preservatives whose usage is prohibited. The compounds that wood smoke leaves behind in meat are of a particularly disagreeable character, and regular consumption of them might theoretically cause considerable harm.

Any thorough investigation of the food-preservative issue always highlights the need for more experimentation and observation. At this time, we are unsure of the effects that long-term intake of food preserved with a certain chemical will have on people of all ages and physical abilities.

I believe there is only one way to learn the truth about the numerous chemicals that have been used to preserve food, and that is to test them out and monitor the outcomes.

To test them properly, on a large enough scale, and for a long enough period of time, however, is a task that cannot be handled by private investigators. This is because we can only hope to gather enough data for conclusive judgments by using it continuously for many years under competent supervision and control. Work of this kind needs to be done and may very easily be done at significant government facilities, such as, for instance, among certain types of prisoners. Although I have no idea how many life or long-term inmates there are, there must be a ton of them. They would make better test subjects for a chemical like boric acid than kids. They represent a group of people whose way of life is fundamentally consistent and whose health records might readily be retained for a lengthy period of years, not because they are prisoners whose destiny or health is of relatively little significance. I am fully aware that my approach would come across to many people as cruel and savage, but compared to the unrecorded boric acid studies that manufacturers have conducted on all different types and conditions of individuals, this experiment would be light and humanitarian. It is regrettable that prisoners are unable to contribute in any way to society. Not many people would likely agree to participate in lengthy feeding trials comparable to the brief ones. If extra incentives were required, a reduced period of service would likely appeal to a large number of people. Furthermore, the argument that putting the health of a small number of men in danger for the benefit of all mankind is stupid given that every civilized nation is willing to sacrifice thousands of its most virulent citizens for the honor of its flag (and its foreign trade) is stupid.

Up until that time, we would be wise to err on the side of caution. The statistics previously mentioned on the higher mortality rates in our country's older age groups impress upon us the need to adopt this approach. Despite what we now know to the contrary, the use of irritant chemical compounds in food may contribute to the relatively high mortality rates from degenerative changes in the kidneys, blood vessels, and other organs.

Even though no single chemical—in the amounts that it is typically present in food—can be reasonably accused of causing serious and long-lasting harm, the total burden placed on the excretory and other organs may be noticeably too high when its effect is multiplied by the effects of other poisonous ingredients found in spiced, smoked, and preserved foods of all kinds. There is no way around the fact that there is a greater chance of negative effects on public health the more extensively and widely preservatives are used in food.

The same category also includes the use of expired or decayed food. It cannot be expected that the unpleasant ingredients created in food by certain types of breakdown may be taken continuously without consequence. We don't even know whether the breakdown products themselves aren't more harmful overall than any possible preservatives that may be applied!

According to what we already know, efforts should thus be focused on

1. Distributing food as fresh as possible and
2. Avoiding any chemical preservatives other than those that have been conclusively shown to be safe. The techniques of food preservation such as drying, cooling, heating, and sealing are supported by both theoretical and practical

evidence. The same can be said for the use of salt and sugar solutions. But from the perspective of public health, the use of sulfites in sausage and chopped meat, the addition of formaldehyde to milk, and the addition of boric acid or sodium fluoride to butter are all practices that should be avoided.

The answer is simple and has been put forward often: pass legislation making it illegal to add any chemical to food unless absolutely necessary. The assumption would therefore be—as it is in fact—that such substances are more or less harmful, and evidence of their safety is required before any particular substance can be labeled as an exception to the general rule. Such regulations would cover the use of substances to "improve the appearance" of meals as well as the use of chemicals or preservatives. As has previously been mentioned, the foolish habit of artificially coloring food results in waste and sometimes dangerous situations. It is not based on any fundamental human need; natural, undisturbed food may become fashionable just as readily as a fashion merchant can change the color and style of apparel. A national panel of experts or a reputable organization like the American Public Health Association should establish the necessary list of exceptions (substances like sugar and salt), which should be subject to a general prohibition on the incorporation of any chemical substance into food for preservative or cosmetic purposes.

FOOD ALTERNATIVES

Sometimes familiar, natural food items are substituted or added to for reasons of economics or convenience by manufactured chemical products or by substances whose food value is less well established. I just need to quickly mention those infamous cases of adulteration, such as the addition of chicory to coffee, powdered olive stones to pepper, or glucose to confectionery. Even if some of these procedures may be unethical in terms of public morality, they cannot be criticized only on sanitary grounds. Chicory is less likely to injure the human body than caffeine, and sprinklings of crushed cocoanut shell are healthier than pepper, as may be claimed with some plausibility. However, there is another category of situations in which artificial replacement is categorically unacceptable. One example is the use of the sweetening agent saccharin, which is made from coal tar. This chemical, whose sweetening power is 500 times greater than that of cane sugar, has no nutritional benefit in the amounts that would be taken, and even small amounts (over 0.3 grams per day) are likely to cause digestive disturbances. It is not a suitable substitute for sugar in everyday meals.

Another well-known example of replacement is the use of inexpensive chemically produced tastes like "fruit ethers" in "soft drinks," fruit syrups, and the like in lieu of the more costly real fruit extracts. The creation of "foam" in "soda water" by saponin, a chemical known to harm red blood cells, is probably more significant hygienically.

There are several additional well-known instances of food replacement, complexity, and adulteration, some of which have clear sanitary drawbacks and others whose only flaw is straightforward deceit. From the perspective of public policy, it can be claimed that almost all of them are inadmissible since they are founded on the desire to misrepresent the nature of foods.

Some people who have carefully tracked the development of food adulteration believe that although overall sophistication—both legally permitted and otherwise—has significantly grown in recent years, the percentage of very harmful adulteration has decreased. Whatever the case, it is obvious that the chance for widespread experimentation with novel drugs should not be left unchecked in the hands of makers and dealers who are primarily driven by financial interests. A tiny number of dishonest people will continue to add cheap, subpar, and sometimes harmful additives to foodstuffs as long as the desire for profit is given free rein. It is necessary to continually tighten the net of limitations. The three main reasons for food tampering are:

1. A desire to prevent food from spoiling or deteriorating;

2. A puerile fantasy—often skillfully fostered for mercenary purposes—for a conventional appearance, as for polished rice, bleached flour, and grass-green peas; and

3. A deliberate attempt to deceive consumers into thinking that something is more valuable than it actually is. Only the first purpose may be said to have any genuine basis, and as previously said, the use of chemical preservatives to satisfy this goal is fraught with sanitary issues and uncertainties. The risks of gradual poisoning from chemically treated foods must be viewed as

equally serious from an impartial perspective on human physiology, despite the fact that they are sneaky and difficult to detect.

CHAPTER FIVE

PATHOGENIC FOOD-BORNE BACTERIA

Pathogenic bacteria are a major cause of many occurrences of 'toxic food,' since they are present in the food. When symptoms appear so quickly after eating, as they do in the usual meat poisoning outbreaks, the specific meal is instantly suspected and examined. In other situations, it is difficult to identify the offending dietary item. Although eating food contaminated with tubercle bacilli likely contributes to certain instances of TB, the exact source and timing of the infection are seldom, if ever, clear.

When pathogenic bacteria are found in food, it is often either because they were introduced by diseased humans when the meal was being prepared or served or because the animal that provided the food was contaminated. In various illnesses, the relative weight of these two components varies greatly.

TYPE 1 FOODBORNE ILLNESS

Since the typhoid bacillus does not affect domestic animals, human contamination is the main factor in all cases of food-borne typhoid. A notable example of food-borne typhoid infection was documented in 1914 in Hanford, California, when consuming Spanish spaghetti given at a community meal resulted in 93 instances of the illness. According to an investigation, the lady who made this meal was a typhoid carrier and was harboring live typhoid bacilli when she combined the sauce for the spaghetti before baking. Additional laboratory testing revealed that the typical oven temperature used to cook the spaghetti was not only insufficient to sterilize the dish but also provided an ideal environment for the bacteria already within the mass to grow. As a result, there was a significant foodborne illness outbreak that affected a sizable majority (57%) of the diners

The adventures of typhoid carrier Mary Malloy, who pursued a career as a chef in and around New York City, are deservedly famous. It is known that Malloy was responsible for at least seven typhoid outbreaks in different houses where she worked, as well as one significant hospital epidemic.

It is very unusual for personnel of restaurants and other public institutions to get typhoid from contaminated food, demonstrating the need to guard against food contamination throughout the whole preparation and serving process. In accordance with this premise, the New York City Department of Health has begun a thorough investigation of the nearly 90,000 chefs and servers who work in the city's public eating establishments. Results in finding typhoid carriers and instances of communicable illness have been achieved, and they adequately support this approach as a crucial step in defending the community against the spread of infection.

Due to their origin, certain foods are more susceptible to typhoid infection than others. Typhoid is more likely to spread via uncooked vegetables like lettuce, celery, radishes, and watercress than from peas, beans, and potatoes. Philadelphia has reported a typhoid epidemic that may be linked to watercress. On June 24, 1913, 43 guests attended a wedding breakfast when watercress sandwiches were provided. Subsequent investigations revealed that 19 of the visitors ate the sandwiches. Within a month, 18 of these people had typhoid fever; the sickness often struck after the visitors had dispersed to their summer residences. Non-consumers of watercress sandwiches were unaffected. Uncooked celery has also been linked to typhoid illness.

In certain cases, the practice of utilizing human waste as fertilizer in truck gardens results in harmful soil pollution that is transmitted to the developing plants and lasts for a very long time.

Vegetables need to be thoroughly washed in order to be bacterially clean. If the rising use of this type of soil enrichment is not immediately stopped, the threat this source poses to the community is likely to worsen in the future.

Typhoid cases in South Philadelphia were on the rise in 1915, which prompted the state health authorities to look into the situation. The bulk of the instances were found to be concentrated in and around three public marketplaces, as was shown by this.

These are all street marketplaces where everything is thrown on sidewalks and pushcarts without any concern for hygienic practices, including fruits, vegetables, pastries, apparel, and random items of every sort. The exposed commodities are handled and picked over by the customers of these marketplaces, increasing the risk of disease transmission.

The Christian Street Market area nearby had the highest concentration of incidents. Residents of the "Little Italy" neighborhood make up the majority of the customers at this market. The majority of shoppers in the South Street Market are Hebrews, but the majority of shoppers at the Seventh Street Market are Poles and Hebrews.

Regarding the relatively high number of instances among people of one nationality, the following conclusion was drawn:

Our inspectors have discovered that the varied techniques employed by Italians and Hebrews to prepare their food are to blame for the higher number of cases discovered in the area of Little Italy's Christian Street Market. While the Hebrews prepare a larger portion of their meals, the Italians like to consume numerous fruits and vegetables fresh. The fact that the inhabitants of the Italian colony have suffered more than the other district residents is probably a result of this tradition.

The typhoid bacillus was discovered on some celery after several vegetables from pushcarts and street marketplaces were analyzed for germs. In such situations, it would naturally be difficult to identify whether the infection resulted from careless handling or came from typhoid bacilli found in the soil where the celery was cultivated.

When sold unwrapped, bread is vulnerable to infection from insects and dirty handling. According to research by Katherine Howell, uncovered loaves of bread sold in Chicago were more or less densely coated with germs and had a substantially higher average number of bacteria than wrapped loaves. Typhoid fever has sometimes been linked directly to bread. Seven cases of typhoid have been reported by Hinton at the Elgin (Illinois) State Hospital. These cases are thought to have been brought on by a typhoid carrier whose job it was to slice the bread before serving. Typhoid cases disappeared once the typhoid-carrying employee was moved to a different department where she handled no raw food.

Foods like milk, which are often consumed uncooked and are therefore conducive to the formation of typhoid bacilli, need to be protected especially well. It is remarkable that a significant decline in the occurrence of typhoid fever has coincided with the mandatory pasteurization of milk in New York, Chicago, and other major American cities. Milk-borne typhoid was a frequent cause of typhoid outbreaks in the United States up until recent years, and this source has been identified in hundreds of cases.

One food animal, the oyster, which is widely consumed raw, has been strongly linked to several typhoid epidemics. However, there haven't been many well-documented outbreaks of oyster typhoid, and the threat from this source has sometimes been overstated. The sewage pollution of the shellfish beds or the brackish water where the oyster is sometimes put to "fatten" before it is sold is the cause of oyster contamination. Oysters, as well as clams and mussels, must be constantly protected against sewage contamination, but the actual occurrence of oyster infection is currently thought to be relatively rare. In recent years, state and federal oversight of the oyster industry in the United States has largely eliminated the taking of oysters from infected waters.

Investigating every case of typhoid fever and tracing it to its source as much as is practical is probably the most efficient way to avoid typhoid food contamination. Typhoid-carriers might be identified using this method, and other infection hotspots could also be identified. Typhoid carriers who are inclined to act against advice can be completely controlled, but this is a challenging challenge that public health authorities have not yet resolved. Once carriers are discovered, they can be given the right guidance and cautioned that they represent a risk to others.

AFRICAN CHOLERA

Domestic animals are not vulnerable to Asiatic cholera, similar to typhoid fever, and all occurrences of illness have a human origin. Food-borne outbreaks of cholera are far less frequent than those of typhoid fever, even in places where the illness is prevalent and usually spreads through contaminated drinking water.

There have been isolated cases of Asiatic cholera that have been linked to tainted milk, fruits, or lettuce; however, these cases are rare and cannot be used as an example of how the illness is typically disseminated. The following experience of the

English bacteriologist Hankin, however, demonstrates the degree to which residents of tropical countries—and perhaps of all lands—are at the mercy of their domestic staff. I've seen a chef chill a jelly by setting it in a little irrigation ditch that ran in front of his cookhouse, the man claims. This sewer was filled with water that originated from a well where I had found the cholera bacteria. He used a spoon to stir the jelly after cleaning it by dipping it in the drain and wiping it with his fingers.

TUBERCULOSIS

Animal studies have shown the transmission of tuberculosis via meat and milk from infected animals. It is still debatable to what extent eating these foods in today's society poses a risk to humans. It is feasible to tell the difference between illnesses in humans brought on by the so-called human tubercle bacillus and infections brought on by the tubercle bacillus of bovine origin by carefully studying the differences between the two.

Additional comparison studies in this area are required and may ultimately allow us to determine the scope of human tuberculosis infection originating from bovine sources more thoroughly than is now achievable.

Because it is seldom consumed raw, meat is a less probable source of illness than milk. The real frequency of TB transmission via the flesh of tuberculous cattle has been highly disputed in the past, and opinions today must still be supported by circumstantial evidence. The use of tuberculous cattle's meat has never been shown to cause human infection. The finding that tubercle bacilli may pass through the intestinal wall undetected and can go to the lungs or other distant organs where they find opportunities for development, however, lessens the relevance of this information. This makes it particularly difficult to get reliable proof, along with the length of time that often elapses between the actual incidence of an illness and the finding that an infection exists.

The fact that the tubercle bacillus is not frequently or abundantly present in the masses of muscle that are typically marketed as "meat," that the tubercle germ itself is not a spore-bearer and is killed by routine cooking, and that reported cases of the finding of tubercle bacilli of bovine origin in adults over the age of sixteen are extremely rare all work against any very frequent occurrence of meat-borne tuberculosis.

This latter point is likely the most compelling proof that, although theoretically feasible, tuberculous meat infection is, at the very least, not frequent. When tuberculous lesions are generalized, extensive in one or both body cavities, "multiple, acute, and actively progressive," or when they are "multiple, acute, and actively progressing," the entire carcass of an animal should be condemned, according to the majority of commissions and official agencies that have thought about the precautions to be taken against a potential tuberculous meat infection. Obviously, any organ displaying tuberculous lesions is not to be consumed as food. On the other hand, if the tuberculous lesion is localized and confined and the major body part is intact, it is thought that pieces of properly examined animals may be sold; in such circumstances, contamination of the meat with dressing must be avoided. The widespread consensus is that when such precautions are followed, the risk of contracting tuberculosis from properly cooked meat is so small as to be insignificant.

Compared to meat, milk is a considerably more probable source of TB transmission. Particularly if the udder is afflicted, freshly extracted raw milk from tuberculous calves may contain vast quantities of tubercle bacilli. The dung of cows with tuberculosis may also contaminate milk. Market milk has been reported to contain tubercle bacilli in varied levels by observers in England, Germany, France, and the United States, and it has been shown that such milk is contagious for lab animals. Although it may be very difficult to trace any specific case of TB to its source, as was said with regard to meat infection, there are other cases in the historical record where the circumstantial evidence clearly suggests that milk was the vehicle of infection.

MILK-BORNE INFECTIONS OF MANY KINDS

According to the information provided in the sections above, milk has the highest risk of introducing disease-causing microorganisms into a person's body out of all meals. This is partially because milk is occasionally obtained from sick animals and partially because, unless great care is taken, it may easily become contaminated during collection and transportation. If milk is ever contaminated with harmful bacteria, these can grow rapidly due to the excellent culture medium it provides. Additionally, it's partially due to the fact that uncooked milk is often consumed. For these reasons, the number of illnesses linked to raw milk greatly outweighs those linked to any other kind of food.

There are a number of illnesses that may spread via milk but are almost never caused by other meals. Among them, diphtheria and scarlet fever are perhaps the most well-known. Even if other types of interpersonal interaction also play a significant role in the spread of both illnesses, certain milk supplies have been consistently linked to the development of both. Scarlet fever and diphtheria that are transmitted via milk seem to be typically, if not always, caused by direct human-source contamination of the milk.

However, some researchers believe that it is feasible for the cow to sometimes get the scarlet fever or diphtheria virus from human sources and occasionally directly contribute to the contamination of the milk.

A serious milk-borne illness known as "septic sore throat" or "streptococcus sore throat," which has recently become noticeable in Boston, Chicago, Baltimore, and other American cities, apparently starts in some cases when an infected milker infects the cow's udder; in other cases, the milk appears to have been directly infected by a human "carrier." It is believed that the exact germ has been identified and that its relationship to the illness has been scientifically proven. Like diphtheria and scarlet fever, this illness may sometimes be acquired by touch. Other than milk, no meal is known to induce it.

Man may get foot-and-mouth disease from diseased cattle by drinking their milk, although it seldom affects people and is generally not particularly dangerous. As far as is known, the only alternative means of transmission to humans is via the consumption of raw milk.

As previously mentioned, the only use of warm milk may help to avoid such instances of infection or "poisoning" by milk. Many doctors believe that the possibility of nutritional problems (like scurvy) in a tiny percentage of children given pasteurized or boiling milk is readily treatable and has a far lower practical value than the prevention of infection.

PROTEUS INFECTION MAY BE POSSIBLE.

Toxic food outbreaks have often been attributed to one widely disseminated microbe known as "Bacillus proteus," but it is still unclear to what extent this charge is true. Although B. proteus and B. coli are related, the majority of these bacteria do not ferment lactose and are considerably more aggressively proteolytic than the latter, as shown by their capacity to liquefy casein and gelatin. They produce gas while fermenting dextrose and producing indol, the same as B. coli. B. proteus species are extensively dispersed in all types of decaying organic waste.

The data supporting the theory that this bacillus is the source of toxic food is not entirely persuasive. The epidemic Pfuhl describes is usual. Four to twelve hours after consuming sausage meat, eighty-one men in a garrison at Hanover were suddenly struck down with severe gastroenteritis. Although the meat was cooked with regular care and was completely normal in terms of look, taste, and smell, it was discovered to have considerable amounts of B. proteus. After the sausage-fed rats and mice became sick, B. proteus was found in their blood and internal organs. However, these animals do sometimes pass away despite being given very regular meat, and after death, B. proteus and other common gut bacteria are often identified from the corpse. In fact, B. proteus is prevalent in many animal feeds as well as in the seemingly healthy human gut.

It commonly infects the internal organs after or just before death, similar to B. coli. Therefore, the presence of B. proteus in food or internal organs does not prove a causal link with certainty. Similar to this, there is conflicting data linking B. proteus infection to other epidemics.

It is also questionable to what extent this species' development of a toxin in food may be held accountable for meat poisoning.

1. Proteus is rather abundant in decaying food, and under certain conditions, it has been seen to produce toxins that are harmful to humans. It's possible that this creature produces hazardous compounds when it first starts to decompose. Mandel and others believe that, if any harmful effects from B. proteus are to be attributed, they are more of an intoxication

than an infection. According to the available data, it's still unclear whether or not this microbe is to blame for toxic food.

INFECTION WITH PARATYPHOIDS

The most typical cases of "toxic food," so to speak, are those in which the symptoms start to show soon after eating and where digestive issues prevail. All severity levels are present in normal group epidemics of this kind, although recovery usually occurs. Modern bacteriological investigations of the vast majority of these cases reveal the presence of bacteria from the so-called paratyphoid group (B. paratyphosus or B. enteritidis). In outbreaks of meat poisoning in particular, paratyphoid bacilli are discovered to be causally connected to them. A list of twenty-seven identical outbreaks in Great Britain as well as forty-two meat poisoning outbreaks in Germany that were proven to include bacilli from this group. Although there have been very few outbreaks of this kind reported in the United States, it cannot be assumed that this is because they are uncommon since toxic food cases are seldom adequately investigated in American communities.

Common paratyphoid outbreaks in an epidemic in Breslau that involved over eighty people, Kaensche reports that chopped beef seemed to be the source of the virus. The animal from which the meat was derived was critically ill (notgeschlachtet), suffering from acute diarrhea and a high temperature. A veterinarian who examined the meat found that it had abnormal conditions in the liver and other organs, deeming it unsuitable for consumption and ordering its destruction. However, it was stolen and smuggled into Breslau, and sections of it were given to other sausage-makers, who mostly marketed it as hamburger steak (Hackfleisch). Nothing unusual about the meat's color, flavor, or firmness could be found. However, after using extremely modest quantities in several situations, disease ensued. Despite some of those affected having really severe symptoms, no one passed away.

Meat was used to isolate bacilli of the Bacillus enteritidis type.

A huge and extremely severe epidemic among the students at a ladies' industrial school in Limerick, Ireland, in November 1908. Out of 197 students, there were 73 instances, and nine of those cases resulted in fatalities. 67 females in the first or Senior class, who ranged in age from thirteen to seventeen, took the brunt of the onslaught. When the 55 females in this class ate beef stew for supper, 53 of them became ill, and eight of them passed away. One of the two who weren't impacted consumed the potatoes and gravy but not the meat. Girls in some of the other courses also consumed some of the allegedly contaminated beef as cold meat, which contributed to their illnesses. A portion of the meat has already been consumed without causing any negative consequences. Either an uneven spread of the virus or thorough cooking that killed it might account for the escape of people who consumed chunks of the same carcass on October 27 and 29 [five days earlier]. However, some of the infectious material must have gotten past the roasting on the 29th and multiplied quickly to make the whole piece very poisonous and infectious during the course of the five days until the fateful Tuesday, when it was eventually ingested. A local butcher had personally butchered the animal from which the forequarter of the steak was taken. No accurate information on the calf's health at the time of slaughter or just before it could be found. However, the meat was offered at such a cheap price that it was clearly not thought to be of the highest quality. The features of the bacilli identified in this epidemic and the agglutination responses of the patient's blood demonstrated that the illness was caused by a typical strain of Bacillus enteritidis.

In July 1915, there was a widespread outbreak of toxic food in and around Westerly, Rhode Island. The epidemic was characterized by the typical signs of severe gastroenteritis, and it was brought on by the consumption of pie from a Westerly restaurant. Everything about the epidemic pointed to a specific batch of pies as the culprit. Sixty people were rendered extremely sick, and four of them died. The pies had nothing peculiar about their flavor or aroma to raise questions. The symptoms appeared after consuming numerous pies created with the identical pie-crust combination, including custard, squash, lemon, chocolate, apple, etc. A pie sample examination led to the isolation of Bacillus paratyphosus B. No clear indication of the precise source of the pie filling contamination was found. Although there had not been a staff turnover for many months, it is conceivable that a paratyphoid carrier brought the pie into the restaurant, which makes this theory completely conjectural. It's possible that an animal-derived substance was the main contaminated component.

Characteristics of a paratyphoid infection generally There are several different paratyphoid food infection symptoms. The first indications of difficulty often occur six to twelve hours after eating, although they may sometimes start as soon as thirty minutes later or take up to forty-eight hours to manifest. Inflammation of the gastrointestinal tract is almost always present and may manifest as minor "indigestion" or mild diarrhea, or it can be quite severe and accompanied by excruciating abdominal pain. Although common, fevers are often not extremely high. Recovery might happen fast, allowing the patient to return to normal within two or three days, or it can happen extremely slowly, leaving the attack's consequences to persist for weeks or months.

Researchers have seen at least two clinical kinds of paratyphoid illness: the more prevalent gastro-intestinal type as described and a second type that often cannot be separated from typhoid fever without rigorous bacterial investigation. It is yet unclear how these two clinical variants relate to the quantity and kind of contaminated food. No variation in paratyphoid bacillus type has been shown to be related to variations in clinical presentation. It's possible that both the quantity and type of toxins and bacteria contained in the meal consumed had an impact. There is little question that the patient's unique quirks play a role.

Despite some ongoing debate on specific paratyphoid infection characteristics, the following key facts have been established:

1. This kind of toxic food is significantly more often linked to certain diet items than to others. The majority of outbreaks that have been documented are linked to eating foods high in

protein, such as meat, milk, fish, and eggs. Fruits have been involved infrequently, but vegetables and grains have been involved less often.

2. It has been shown that the meat in question came from an animal that was killed while ill (_notgeschlachtet_, to use the expressive German phrase). However, this is not the case in all instances of paratyphoid meat poisoning. It would seem reasonable to assume that in an animal that was "killed to save its life," the particular paratyphoid germ was present as an illness prior to death. Additionally, milk has been linked to paratyphoid poisoning, and in some of these instances, it was discovered that the milk came from a cow that had enteritis or another condition.

3. There is evidence that initially healthy food can become contaminated with paratyphoid bacilli during preparation or serving in the same way

that it can become contaminated with typhoid bacilli; this is frequently caused by a paratyphoid carrier handling the food. The illness may sometimes spread from person to person; however, this method of transmission looks very uncommon and is much less common than "contact" infection in typhoid.

4. The use of raw or partially cooked food is linked to the majority of paratyphoid epidemics. People who have consumed the allegedly harmful food ingredient raw or improperly prepared are often the ones who suffer the most, whereas others who have consumed it after it has been cooked are left unaffected.

The consumption of meat from a cow that was butchered as a result of having a severe case of enteritis. 58 people were affected in varied degrees of severity; one young worker who consumed roughly 800 grams of raw meat died as a consequence of the incident. A bacillus with the designation. In addition to the cow's flesh and intestines, It was discovered via vaccination studies that it was pathogenic for a variety of animal species. Since then, a number of subsequent meat poisoning episodes in Germany, Belgium, France, and England have yielded bacilli with characteristics comparable to these. The paratyphoid bacillus has been implicated in one well-documented case of toxic food in the United States.

The paratyphoid group of bacteria is closely related to the actual typhoid bacillus, but they differ from that organism in that they can ferment glucose while producing gas. They are less highly pathogenic for humans but more highly pathogenic for lower animals than the typhoid bacillus. When injected into milk containing a few drops of litmus, the majority of paratyphoid bacilli types that cause toxic food release a significant quantity of alkali more or less quickly over time. This causes the milk to eventually take on a deep blue hue. There are several different types of paratyphoid bacilli that have been identified. These kinds of primary variations are agglutinative differences. This means that certain culturally related paratyphoid bacteria discovered in connection with additional outbreaks will not agglutinate in the blood serum of an animal that has been inoculated with a particular culture or strain, but will agglutinate that culture and other strains isolated from specific other meat poisoning epidemics. No consistent differentiation between these variations has been shown to exist, with the exception of this one instance of an agglutination response. The clinical characteristics of the infections caused by the various kinds in humans and other animals seem to be quite similar, if not identical.

Gärtner's bacillus, often known as B. enteritidis or Gärtner's bacillus, was first identified by Gärtner (loc. cit.) and is typically thought to be one of the agglutinative variants. In several locations in Germany and Belgium, outbreaks of meat poisoning have been linked to bacteria that exhibit every characteristic of Gärtner's bacillus. Mayer has prepared a record of forty-eight occurrences of toxic food that were attributable to B. enteritidis Gärtner These outbreaks resulted in around 2000 illnesses and 20 fatalities. Twenty-three of the forty-eight outbreaks included meat from animals that were known to be unwell at the time of the slaughter or just before it. Eleven of the remaining twenty-five breakouts were brought on by sausage and chopped meat of unknown origin. One of the B. enteritidis outbreaks and two others were linked to potato salad and vanilla pudding, respectively.

In some cases of toxic food, a bacillus that is culturally related to the Gärtner bacillus is discovered, but it will not agglutinate with the Gärtner bacillus serum. The bacilli discovered in human instances of paratyphoid fever, which are not known to be related to toxic food, exhibit almost comparable culture and agglutination responses to those of this strain. 77 cases of food-related illness were attributed to various species known as "B. suipestifer" were believed to be the cause. Two thousand cases in all and twenty fatalities are almost equal to those linked to B. enteritidis. Meat from animals that are unquestionably ill is less often linked to outbreaks of this kind (ten in seventy-seven) than B. enteritidis outbreaks (twenty-three in forty-eight), according to Mayer's tabulation. However, 18 cases were linked to sausage and chopped meat of unknown origin.

The "B. suipestifer" bacillus is currently believed to be just a secondary invader in hog cholera. It is identical to the bacillus known as "B. paratyphosus" B in its cultural and, to a large extent, in its agglutinative behavior, but some researchers believe that it can be distinguished from the latter on the basis of particularly delicate discriminatory tests. The real instances of toxic food, according to Bainbridge, Savage, and other English researchers, should be attributed to the bacterium known as B. suipestifer. These researchers would reserve the label "B. paratyphosus" for bacteria that cause "an illness clinically indistinguishable from typhoid fever." German researchers, however, believe that B. suipestifer and B. paratyphosus B are one and the same. My own research suggests that there is a significant difference between these two groups.

The debate about the location of the bacteria that cause toxic food in nature directly relates to this question. The majority of researchers in Germany, where the majority of toxic food outbreaks have occurred or at least been bacteriologically studied, believe that B. suipestifer (also known as B. paratyphosus B) is much more widely distributed than B. enteritidis and that it occurs quite frequently in the intestinal tract of healthy people, especially in certain regions, like the southern part of the German Empire. It is believed that these paratyphoid carriers may contaminate food during handling or preparation, much as typhoid carriers are known to do. Jacobitz and Kayser (vermicelli), Reinhold (fish), and others have recorded a number of incidents where it is believed that food contamination during preparation occurred. In one incident, according to Reinhold, many people who had cared for the sick people had become ill themselves, suggesting a probable contact infection. Reinhold also noted that in another incident, people who had the contaminated food—in this instance, dried codfish—on the first day did not have the same level of illness as those who consumed the leftovers on the second day. Patients' feces were used to isolate a bacillus from the paratyphoid group but not from dried codfish. These facts were understood to mean that the bacilli increased in the meal while it was standing and that the fish had gotten contaminated during the cooking procedure.

There is no question that certain instances of paratyphoid toxic food are brought on by tainted food that was prepared, or at the very least, by human carriers of the virus. According to the majority of English bacteriologists and many German investigators, the bacilli in such instances are typically or invariably of the B. suipestifer type. Other instances are caused by pathogenic bacteria that are obtained from sick animals, and these bacteria (B. enteritidis Gärtner) often, if not always, have a slightly different nature. It is currently unclear whether the two kinds of toxic food bacteria are constantly linked to human or animal disease processes or if they are just widely distributed organisms that sometimes exhibit harmful traits. Such bacteria are seldom, if ever, identified in certain areas, such as North Germany and England, unless they are linked to specific instances of sickness. On the other hand, they are said to happen extraordinarily often in the intestines of healthy humans and animals in several areas of Southwest Germany. According to Savage, the development of saprophytic bacteria known as "Paragaertner" forms, which closely resemble the "true" Gärtner bacilli, has led to some misunderstanding on this issue. Only after a lengthy battery of tests can they be separated from each other. The bacilli in this category exhibit amazing variety, and according to some researchers, sometimes "mutations" take place that change one kind into another.

Despite the current ambiguity around the link and relevance of the observed variants, the following facts stand out clearly in the chaos:

1. The majority of cases of meat poisoning that have been bacterially examined in recent years may be linked to one or more members of this group and not to "ptomain poisoning."
2. When consumed with food, bacteria belonging to the _paratyphoid enteritidis_ group that are culturally similar but agglutinatively distinct may cause the same clinical signs in humans.
3. When these bacteria are directly isolated from sick animals, they are more likely to be of the Gärtner type (B. enteritidis) than the Suipestifer type.

GENERATION OF TOXINS

The issue of this type of bacteria producing a toxin and its potential link to toxic food have received a lot of attention. A soluble toxin is present in broth cultures that have had the live bacilli killed by heat or eliminated by filtering. When mice, guinea pigs, or rabbits are injected with this sterile soup, the animals die as a result. The only thing that is essentially known about the hazardous compounds in question is that they are heat-resistant. Since there is no proof that they cause the development of antibodies when administered to sensitive animals, they are most likely not to be classified with the so-called genuine toxins produced by the diphtheria and tetanus bacilli. Some researchers believe that the formation of these toxic bodies by the paratyphoid-enteritidis bacilli in meat and other protein foodstuffs is to blame for some outbreaks as well as some toxic food phenomena. The rapid onset of symptoms is thought to be caused by the ingested poisons, whereas the later manifestations are thought to be those of a true infection. The fact that well-prepared food has been shown to be noticeably less likely to induce toxic food than raw or improperly cooked food is in opposition to this viewpoint.

The main causes of meat poisoning outbreaks that have been documented include meat pies, puddings, and jellies, as well as sausages manufactured from raw meat. This is most likely because the heat required to prepare these items does not sufficiently kill germs. It is interesting that raw milk consumers are the ones that are impacted by epidemics that are milk-borne. For instance, it is reported that there is a significant B. enteritidis epidemic in and around Newcastle, England:

Nobody who had solely consumed boiling milk was ever known to have had an issue. So, in one household, which included a husband, wife, and the woman's mother, the two ladies drank a modest amount of farm-fresh raw milk—no more than a tumblerful—and both became unwell approximately twelve hours later. On the other hand, the husband typically drank one pint each day, but he always boiled it. In this particular instance, he behaved normally and was unfazed.

The claim that a heat-resistant toxin is present in such situations is not conclusive when it is also taken into account that routine roasting or broiling of a piece of meat is often not adequate to achieve a germicidal temperature throughout. Additionally, it should be noted that in some outbreaks, people who consumed raw or partially cooked meat became ill, while people who consumed well-cooked meat from the same animal remained unaffected. This would seem to indicate that living bacilli were destroyed by heat, as the toxic compounds these organisms produce are heat-resistant. The idea that a specific infection takes place is further supported by the fact that the paratyphoid bacillus is usually agglutinated by the blood serum of infected individuals. If only harmful chemicals were to blame for the symptoms, this wouldn't be the case. Overall, it is impossible to say what role the toxins produced by B. enteritidis and its friends play in food consumed outside of the body. According to the information available, the majority, if not the only, way that the bacilli in this category are dangerous is through infection.

ORIGINS OF THE INFECTION

The two primary causes of Enteritidis-suipestifer infection are:

1. Ill domestic animals, whose contaminated meat or milk is consumed; and
2. Human carriers who infect food while it is being prepared or served. A third option may be added to these:
3. Food being contaminated by bacteria from this category, which are common in the intestines of healthy animals Think about things in this order:

1. **Diseased animals**: Meat from pigs or cattle accounts for the bulk of instances of meat poisoning. There have also been sporadic

outbreaks linked to eating rabbit, sheep, geese, fish, shrimp, and oysters. The relative rarity of illnesses caused by eating sheep meat is particularly notable. Regarding the clinical symptoms these bacteria generate in animals and the connection between those disorders and future human infections, more precise knowledge is required. Although it is not currently thought that this bacillus is the cause of hog cholera, it is regularly seen in the swine's internal organs after death and is usually linked to the illness as an accessory or secondary invader. Human infections could be expected to be more frequent than in other districts in areas where hog cholera is rampant; however, this does not seem to be the case. Although B. suipestifer is known to be extensively distributed in hog cholera outbreaks, the so-called "B. suipestifer infections" in humans have never been connected to such outbreaks. Use of the flesh or milk of the infected animals has resulted in poisoning due to suppurative processes in cattle, particularly calves. It has been repeatedly shown that bacteria belonging to the _enteritidis-suipestifer_ group cause intestinal disturbances, including symptoms like "calf diarrhea," as well as udder inflammation in cows, a variety of septicemic conditions in cattle, and other domestic animals. It has previously been highlighted how often people have been ill after eating meat from "emergency-slaughtered" animals. The infection-causing strain was found in the cardiac blood of a cow that had passed away with contagious diarrhea.

2. **Human contamination**: There is some evidence that in certain cases of paratyphoid food illnesses, the food was initially produced from a healthy animal but acquired the disease through human sources during the preparation process. But the evidence in this instance is not quite convincing. Söderbaum refers to a milk-borne

paratyphoid outbreak that occurred in Kristiania and was blamed on a female milker infecting the milk. A fascinating paratyphoid epidemic affecting 19 out of 250 soldiers in a military corps. The individuals developed illnesses on various days. It was discovered that an assistant chef who had been working in the kitchen for many months had been affected by a mild illness that was not yet definitively recognized just before the epidemic eruption.

After being admitted to the hospital, he was given a convalescent release. After being recalled and placed under quarantine, the chef admitted that he had been ill with a headache and anorexia a few days . Nevertheless, he had kept up his work in the kitchen. Later B. paratyphosus B (B. suipestifer) was consistently discovered in his stools. Therefore, it is most likely that the epidemic was brought on by food tainted by a paratyphoid carrier who had undergone a failed feverish attack.

An outbreak of acute gastro-enteritis that occurred in a boarding house. It was discovered that not one food item had been consumed by all of the affected individuals, and there were other reasons to suspect that the outbreak was caused by a servant who was a carrier of a variety of food contamination.

Therefore, there is reason to think that bacteria from this category, which are derived from human sources, may occasionally contaminate food. However, it is unclear how often this form of infection occurs in comparison to infections that come from sick animals. It must also be acknowledged that English researchers have a tendency to classify epidemics similar to those just described as infections with B. paratyphosus B, a microorganism they would differentiate from the "true" toxic food bacilli, B. enteritidis and B. suipestifer.

3. **Other contaminations**: According to certain researchers, particularly some German authors, the paratyphoid group of bacilli is so extensively dispersed in nature that trying to stop the illness from spreading is like trying to stop a windmill. This point of view contends that bacilli are regularly found in our daily environments and thus find their way into a range of meals on a regular basis. Intestinal paratyphoid bacilli have been found by a number of German researchers in the intestines of animals that seemed healthy, including pigs, cattle, rats, and mice, as well as more infrequently other species, in water and ice, German sausage, and chopped meat, and in the bodies of persons who appeared to be in good condition. It has yet to be shown to what degree the purported ubiquity of

these organisms is attributable to incorrect bacterial identification, as some English researchers have asserted. Without a doubt, there are certain places where inflated ideas about the actual paratyphoid bacteria's widespread prevalence have persisted. Savage and others think it's completely unreasonable to assume that episodes of toxic food are caused by routine fecal contamination of food. It is argued that there is solid evidence supporting the frequent presence of intestinal bacteria in foods like sausages and chopped meat and that if paratyphoid infections could result from routine intestinal bacterial contamination unrelated to any particular animal infection, toxic food outbreaks would instead be exceedingly common as opposed to being relatively uncommon as they currently are.

Even those who continue to insist that these bacilli are prevalent acknowledge that there are certain locations where they are more abundant than others. For instance, it seems that there are a sizable number of paratyphoid bacilli in southwest Germany. The inconsistencies between German and British researchers' reported results may be explained by regional variations in distribution.

The association of these bacilli with rats and mice is a unique scenario. The so-called Danysz bacillus, one of the many bacteria of the paratyphoid group, is very dangerous for rats and is sometimes utilized as a "rat virus" in different forms for rodent eradication. According to more or less convincing evidence, a number of outbreaks of toxic food in humans have been linked to food being contaminated by one of these viruses, either intentionally, as in the case described by Shibayama, where men ate cakes meant for rats, or inadvertently, through the consumption of mice or rats that have been exposed to the virus. Since the animals may continue to carry the virus' bacilli and spread them on or near food items after seeming to recover, the use of such viruses in rodent control has not been shown to be of very large practical utility and is subject to major hygienic problems.

It is plausible that without human involvement, some bacteria in this group may infect rats and mice and that these afflicted animals could then contaminate food, leading to epidemics of toxic food. Naturally, obtaining evidence of how often this really happens is challenging.

There is no way to avoid the conclusion that the precise source of infection in any one episode of toxic food is often highly conjectural.

Even when there is a strong suspicion regarding a specific food item, it may not be possible to prove beyond a reasonable doubt whether the ingredient (meat or milk) originated from a diseased animal or whether it contracted the disease from other sources (people or other animals) at some point during the preparation and serving process. The instances that can be definitively linked to food obtained from an ill animal are those that have been documented most often.

PREVENTION STRATEGIES

The establishment of an inspection system that will keep as much material from diseased animals off the market as is practical is the most visible and likely most significant approach to avoiding infection with paratyphoid bacilli. Such an inspection must focus on looking at the live animal to be most effective. Diseased animals' milk or meat often lacks outward signs of abnormalities. The veterinary surgeon who was in charge of inspecting the slaughterhouse during the Ghent epidemic of 1895 was so certain that the meat he had cleared could not have been related to the outbreak that he consumed several portions to prove its safety. The experiment had a fatal outcome since the inspector soon developed severe cholera symptoms and passed away five days later. Paratyphoid bacilli were discovered during the postmortem. Müller also recounted a situation in which paratyphoid bacilli were discovered in meat that had caused a meat poisoning epidemic, despite the fact that the flesh had a normal look and the animal's organs exhibited no outward signs of illness. It is clear that examination of a live animal often reveals illness signs that may go undetected during routine screening of slaughterhouse products.

Although it is crucial to examine milking cows and food animals before slaughter, this does not provide total safety. It must be emphasized again and again that even meat and, in particular, milk from animals that seem to be in good condition may have paratyphoid bacilli. Direct bacterial inspection of the corpses of slain food animals has been suggested as a partial solution to this problem, although it appears barely workable as a comprehensive solution. Despite all the safety measures performed at the time of slaughter, it is likely that sometimes meat contaminated with paratyphoid will get past the first line of defense and end up on the market.

This risk, which under a reasonable system of live animal inspection is probably not very serious, may be mitigated by fully boiling all animal-derived meals. Notably, certain internal organs, such as the liver and kidneys, are more likely to contain germs than the vast quantities of muscle that are often consumed as "meat." Due to their makeup and method of preparation, sausages and chopped meat (commonly known as "hamburger steak") should also be handled carefully.

Raw sausage and sick goose liver (paté de foie gras) are examples of foods that carry a comparatively significant risk. The chance of problems is significantly reduced by thorough boiling of food, as is true of most other types of toxic food.

It is apparent that general measures of care and cleanliness will be more or less a precaution regardless of the particular degree of threat from food contamination by healthy paratyphoid carriers (man or domestic animals). Similar to typhoid fever, all paratyphoid epidemics should be extensively researched in order to identify and eradicate the infection's causes. The potential link between these outbreaks and rats and mice should serve as another motivation to control the population of these pests and implement measures to safeguard food against their intrusion.

CHAPTER SEVEN

PET PARASITES

In addition to dangerous bacteria, the human body may sometimes get infected by certain animal parasites that live on or in food. Trichiniasis's parasite is one of the most significant of them.

TRICHINIASIS

Trichiniasis, also known as trichinosis, is a condition marked by fever, muscle aches, a significant increase in eosinophil blood corpuscles, and other more or less well-defined symptoms. At first, typhoid fever is occasionally mistaken for trichiniasis by medical professionals. The parasite at fault is a roundworm called Trichinella spiralis (formerly known as Trichina), which is ingested when in the encysted larval stage in raw or unevenly cooked pork. The digestive juices disintegrate the cysts or envelopes that the parasites are living in, and the immature larvae that are released grow in the small intestine to become the adult worm, generally within two days. The immature embryos, which are generated in large quantities by the adult worms, enter the lymphatic system and bloodstream and, after approximately ten days, start to invade the muscles, which causes many of the infection's most recognizable symptoms. According to estimates, severe instances might result in the circulation of up to fifty million embryos. The symptoms often progressively go away when the parasites eventually stop acting up and encrusting the muscular tissue. When several parasites are consumed at once, it often has devastating consequences; trichiniasis, for example, has a death rate that is typically just over 5% but may reach 30% during severe outbreaks. However, a lot of infections are so small as to go undetected. discovered Trichinella embryos in 5.4% of the corpses of people dying of other causes. These results are thought to show that even in the United States, minor Trichinella infections occur often.

This may be anticipated given that pigs are often infected; the parasite was discovered in roughly 6% of these animals.

The specific symptoms of trichiniasis, such as the muscular pain, may be partly caused by mechanical damage to the muscle tissue, but it is also likely that these symptoms are partially caused by toxic substances secreted by the worms and partially by the introduction of foreign protein material—the worm's protein—into the tissues. Secondary bacterial infection is another option, although there is no evidence that it plays a significant role in the majority of trichiniasis cases. The many stages of the disease's progression are clearly related to the various stages of the worm's growth, including the worm's initial localization in the intestines, invasion of the muscles, and eventual encystment.

Swine may get this parasite by consuming contaminated meat leftovers, their own kind's offal, or infected rats. Because of its propensity for cannibalism, the rat commonly contracts the illness and is a major contributor to its widespread spread. Infection of humans is essentially incidental and self-contained; physiologically, the parasite does not consider humans as hosts when making decisions.

Treatment for an existing trichiniasis infection is palliative rather than completely curative. Once within the body, parasites cannot be significantly impacted by the administration of any medication. Trichiniasis is so difficult, if not impossible, to treat, but it is relatively easy to avoid. All food must be thoroughly cooked in order to prevent infection. Instead of laboriously microscopically examining the tissues of each killed hog, this very easy approach of killing the larvae is a more reliable and affordable method of avoiding infection. Over 32% of the 6,329 instances of trichinosis that were studied in Germany between 1881 and 1898 were linked to meat that had been microscopically inspected and found to be free of trichinae. On the other hand, thorough cooking completely eliminates any risk.

TENIASIS

You may get different tapeworm or cestode illnesses by eating meat that has the parasite in it. Particular tapeworm species, such as Tenia saginata in cattle and Tenia solium in hogs, often infest the flesh of their particular hosts. The dwarf tapeworm, Hymenolepis nana, is developed in rats, and the sporadic human infections with this parasite are likely brought on by these rodents contaminating food.

The presence of tapeworms in humans is occasionally confined to the gastrointestinal tract, with symptoms ranging from mild to severe. However, occasionally (Tenia solium), the larval stage of the tapeworm invades tissues and becomes encrusted in various organs (brain, eye, etc.), with potentially fatal consequences in cases of cerebral infection. Known as "Cysticercus cellulosae," the encysted larva of "Tenia solium" was formerly thought to be a distinct animal species. Because of the presence of this encysted parasite, "measly pork" is a condition.

The so-called hydatid illness is brought on by a cystic growth that the larva of a kind of tapeworm (Echinococcus) that lives in a dog's gut produces. Both contaminated food and, more directly, touching diseased dogs with dirty hands may result in human illness. A variety of tapeworm species that infest fish, particularly certain freshwater species, may enter the human body via raw or partially cooked fish.

The killing of the larvae by heat, or the complete cooking of all meat and fish, as well as minimizing close contact with animals, such as dogs and cats, that are prone to carrying parasites, are methods for preventing tapeworm infection. Cleanliness in food preparation and service, as well as consideration for hand washing before meals and, particularly after handling pets, are required corollaries.

UNCINARIASIS

Although the skin of the feet is the most common site of hookworm infection (uncinariasis, ankylostomiasis), the possibility of a mouth infection cannot be discounted, and in areas where hookworm disease is present, methods of protecting against food contamination should be used, along with other precautions. According to Billings and Hickey, unconscious coprophagy (from raw vegetables) causes hookworm illness considerably more commonly than is widely believed.

ADDITIONAL PARASITES

Other parasitic worms, such as Strongyloides, Ascaris, or eelworm, and Oxyuria, or pinworm, could theoretically infect humans through tainted food. While, as in the case of hookworm disease, other modes of infection are likely more significant, the potential for sporadic infection by uncooked food must not be disregarded.

Giardia (Lamblia) intestinalis infection has been linked to a number of dysentery or diarrheal conditions. It has been shown that certain parasite strains of human origin are harmful to mice and kittens. It is thought that these animals might serve as disease reservoirs and transmit the illness by contaminating human food.

CHAPTER EIGHT

FOOD-BASED POISONS CREATED BY BACTERIA AND OTHER MICRO-ORGANISMS

There are several well-documented examples of toxic food caused by chemicals that have been produced in food while it is still outside the body, which is closely related to the cases of infection with animal or plant parasites that have been addressed. According to popular belief, this is the most prevalent kind of toxic food, but in reality, the cases of this class are far less numerous than those with actual infection with bacteria from the paratyphoid-enteritidis group (chapter vi). Botulism and ergotism are now the most well-known instances of toxicity caused by microorganisms.

ERGOTISM

Ergotism, often known as ergot poisoning, is brought on by the use of rye that has contracted a disease from being contaminated by the fungus

Claviceps purpurea. It happened regularly in the Middle Ages when, in the absence of better food, ergot or spurred rye (O.Fr. _argot, "a cock's spur") was commonly consumed. It is reported that forty thousand people died as a result of this in Limoges in 922. Ergotism is now much less common because of advancements in food transportation infrastructure and the employment of unique techniques for distinguishing contaminated grain from healthy grain in areas where harvests have failed. Hirsch noted around 28 instances of this poisoning in the nineteenth century, but it has essentially stopped in Western Europe. The sickness is reportedly still present in certain regions of Russia after years of poor crop production.

Ergot has long been used as a medication in obstetrics, although its complicated chemical makeup is still poorly understood. It has been discovered that ergot contains a number of elements, each of which has a unique physiological impact. The drug does not completely replicate the symptoms of ergotism outbreaks from medieval times, and it is believed that these symptoms may have been partly caused by the semi-starvation caused by the consumption of rye, from which the fungus had largely removed the nutritious portions.

BOTULISM

The deadly illness known rather erroneously as botulism (botulus, sausage) is the best documented instance of toxic food caused by bacterial products consumed with the meal. Around 1820, the German poet and medical writer Justinus Kerner appears to have been the first to identify and describe this particular kind of toxic food. It features a distinctive set of symptoms. In two publications (1820–22), he lists 174 instances, 71 of which were fatal, that occurred in Württemberg between 1793 and 1822, with the consumption of improperly smoked sausage seeming to be a factor in the majority of cases. Mayer compiles data on 600 further instances that were discovered in different German regions up to the end of 1908, with a total death rate of roughly 25% for the 800 cases. France is said to have extremely few cases of botulism. Savage claims that he has not been able to identify a single outbreak in Great Britain.

On Tuesday, November 23, 1913, a girl of 23 years old ate supper that included light green canned string beans and some rare roast meat. The eyes did feel strained after some stitching around 10:00 in the evening the next day, but she felt completely normal. When the patient awakened on Thursday morning, 36 hours after the meal, her eyes were blurry, her appetite was poor, and she felt very exhausted. She continued to have no appetite at night, felt queasy, and vomited the lunch she had just had. Two and a half days after the meal, on Friday morning, the eyes were worse, items moving quickly were seen twice, and it was noted that the eyes had a propensity to be crossed. There were also complaints of an odd mistiness in the eyes. She didn't leave her bed until late in the afternoon to see Dr. Black. She had previously had some difficulty swallowing, and she described how deglutition felt as though "something came up from below." The fourth day, she stayed in bed, had severe constipation, and observed a significant drop in the volume of urine passed. No headache, no subnormal temperature, and a normal pulse were present, and the only discomfort experienced was the infrequent, minor stomach cramping. On the fourth and fifth days, swallowing was almost impossible, and breathing sometimes got difficult. The patient reported a dry mouth and a bothersome thirst. On the sixth day, there were times when I felt as if I was being suffocated, along with a general sensation of unease and the possibility that I would have trouble breathing. The top lids had started to droop. It was a nasal voice. Liquids that were attempted to be swallowed were returned via the nose. The patient felt noticeably underweight.

Physical examination at this time revealed ptosis of both upper eyelids, a dilated right pupil, a slow response of both pupils to light, apparent paralysis of the internal rectus of the left eye, a normal retina, an inability to raise the head, an apparent loss of control of the neck muscles, an inability to swallow, and a lack of taste. The throat and tongue were both thickly covered in a viscid, yellowish mucus that adhered to the mucosal membrane. Although it could be elevated, the soft palate was slow, especially on the right side. The right tonsil's exudate was so noticeable that it partially resembled a diphtheritic membrane. On the seventh day, there was some improvement in the situation; there were sporadic times when swallowing was easier and there was less of a propensity to strangle. On the eleventh day, the eyes showed some improvement, although they continued to choke while eating. Additionally, the taste buds were more acute, and the overall health was better. The patient could move her head on the twelfth day, but she was unable to raise it until she grabbed her hair braids and dragged them forward. The swallowing was much better, the eyelids could be opened somewhat, and the speech was clearer and less nasal.

After two weeks, the patient was able to eat soft foods without restriction, and after four weeks, she was able to sit up for a few hours without complaining, other than of general weakness and the inability to utilize her eyes. After five weeks, she was allowed to leave the hospital, go back to her house, and eventually start working again.

This kind of food illness always has a significant impact on the neurological system. Dizziness, double vision, trouble swallowing and chewing, as well as other symptoms of nerve involvement, appear in varied degrees of severity and may last for a considerable amount of time after the onset of the attack. Respiration, pulse, and temperature all continue to be essentially normal.

Compared to the typical form of toxic food, gastro-intestinal symptoms may be minimal or nonexistent. Constipation is more common than diarrhea, and there is often minimal stomach discomfort. Vomiting may sometimes happen, but it may not. There was "an entire absence of the usual gastro-intestinal symptoms from first to last, no pain or sensory disturbance, and no elevation of temperature" in the instances that Sheppard documented. The visual distortions are quite recognizable. The following are the experiences Stiles describes:

A few hours after eating, he experienced shocking vertigo and nystagmus—a sense that the automobile taking him to his home was climbing an infinite spiral, that the stars were making circles in the sky, and that the houses along the roadside were reeling. As I was brought inside, the illuminated entryway of my home appeared to come closer and encircle me.

Right now, my bed is just a vertical surface that I can't see serving as a place of rest. Every time I opened my eyes on this day [the next day], the room seemed to be spinning horribly. Eight days after the assault started, even very gently turning my head from one side to the other caused the overwhelming giddiness to worsen. The nystagmus was now only present for brief periods, but in its stead, I noticed an odd diplopia. The picture of one retina was slanted away from parallel by around 15 degrees rather than just being out of alignment with the other. As my recovery progressed, this magnificent diplopia eventually gave way to the more common form, and this happened less and less often. From this day on, my rehabilitation followed a path that was demoralizingly slow but without any setbacks. The indicated visual issues were one of the enduring symptoms. Usually, the left pupil is smaller than the right, and I felt I saw a tiny left-eye accommodation problem. For many weeks, reading was challenging, and writing took longer to resume since it required more focus.

Sheppard noted that visual symptoms were often the earliest indications of a problem, with complaints of double vision, haziness, and difficulty hitting the target while shooting being the most common.

The period of time between consuming the suspect meal and the appearance of the first symptoms is typically twelve to forty-eight hours, although it may be considerably shorter. The gap in Stiles' instance was reportedly less than three hours.

Lesions on the body's tissues In fatal instances, none of the typical gross organ alterations are seen. Some authors have claimed that the so-called Nissl granules, in particular, undergo microscopic degenerative alterations in the ganglion cells. However, in the meticulously examined instance described by Ophüls , the Nissl granules were fairly normal in size, organization, and staining properties. In actuality, there was no evidence to support the idea that the poison had a particular effect on the nerve cells. Ophüls, on the other hand, discovered many thromboses in both the arteries and veins as well as numerous hemorrhages in the brainstem. Therefore, he maintains that the symptoms of botulism poisoning can be explained by signs of severe disturbances in brain circulation associated with hemorrhages and thrombosis in the medulla and pons without resorting to the presumption that the poison has a particular effect on particular ganglion cells.

BACTERIOLOGY

Van Ermengem found that the toxin generated by a bacillus he designated "B. botulinus" is what causes botulism poisoning. In Ellezelles (Belgium), parts of a ham that had been the source of fifty instances of poisoning (1895), as well as the spleen and stomach contents of one of the three fatal cases, were utilized to isolate this bacterium.

The bacillus can only grow in the absence of oxygen (strictly anaerobic); it stains using Gram's technique; it produces terminal spores; and it thrives at a temperature of 22 °C. It seems to be unable to grow in the human body, unlike the majority of bacteria that are harmful to humans, and its harmful effects are only caused by the toxin it produces in foods consumed outside of the body. Botulism is an intoxication rather than an infection. The comparatively infrequent incidence of botulism is at least partially explained by the fact that the bacillus can only thrive in nature when the supply of free oxygen is shut off, since not all of the circumstances required for the creation of the botulinum toxin are often met. Almost little is known about the distribution of B. botulinus. There has only ever been one natural report, with the exception of poisoning incidents. The botulism poison is a true bacterial toxin that is chemically unstable, destroyed by heating to 80°C for 30 minutes, capable of inducing violent symptoms in minute doses, and possessing the property typical of all true toxins of producing an antitoxin when injected into the bodies of susceptible animals in small, non-fatal doses. The toxin produced by B. botulinus has been discovered to be capable of replicating the usual clinical picture of this kind of toxic food in trials on animals. When guinea pigs, rabbits, and other animals get an injection of a filtered broth culture in amounts as little as 0.0001 c.c., paralysis symptoms are induced.

EPIDEMIOLOGY

In general, it appears more likely that the organism is widely distributed but that it does not frequently find favorable conditions for entry into and multiplication in human food. It is possible that there are localities where this bacillus is particularly abundant in the soil or in the intestinal contents of swine or other domestic animals.

Practically every instance of botulism that has been documented has been brought on by food that has had some type of pre-treatment, such as smoking, pickling, or canning, before being left to stand and consumed without further cooking. It is obvious that an uncommon combination of variables must come into play in order for botulism poisoning to occur since both the bacillus, including the spore stage, and its toxin are eliminated by very mild heating. These include, obviously, the following:

1. The presence of the bacilli in sufficient numbers in an appropriate food;
2. The initial preparation of the food by a technique that does not kill the B. botulinus—inadequate smoking, too weak brine, or inadequate cooking;
3. The holding of this inadequately preserved food for a sufficient amount of time under the right conditions of temperature and lack of oxygen; and

4. The use of this food, in which circumstances have conspired to It appears just as logical to assume that the relative rarity of botulism is caused by the rare occurrence of these several circumstances as it is by the rarity of the particular bacillus. The toxic ham in the Belgian epidemic Van Ermengem researched had been at the bottom of a brine cask (anarobic circumstances), whereas the second ham from the same animal had been lying on top of it but was not coated by brine and had been eaten without having any harmful effects. The existence or lack of suitable circumstances for anamorphic development seems to be the deciding factor in this case.

TREATMENT AND PREVENTION

The incriminated ham in the Römer case had bluish-gray patches from which B. botulinus could be separated, but this condition does not seem to have drawn attention before the poisoning and was discovered only after the fact. According to what is known, the meat that has led to botulism has always originated from healthy animals. However, as most anarobes create butyric acid, there is nothing distinctly identifiable about this. In some situations, the implicated food item is reported to have had a rancid or caustic flavor (due to butyric acid?). If the meal (canned beans) is given with salad dressing, as in the Darmstadt and Stanford University outbreaks, a sour flavor may go unnoticed or even enhance the pleasure. Sheppard described a situation in which the canned beans had excellent flavor, aroma, and look.

The first apparent step in preventing this kind of illness is to utilize effective food preservation techniques. According to the reported outbreaks, home-prepared vegetables and meats are more likely to cause botulism than those made in a large-scale commercial kitchen. The major canning facilities' widespread use of steam under pressure offers a high level of protection against anaerobic bacteria and their resistant spores. Any canned or preserved food with an unusual look, taste, or odor should be discarded, regardless of the method of treatment. An additional measure of protection is to promptly reheat any prepared items. Foods like salads that are entirely or partially made of raw ingredients shouldn't be left out overnight before serving.

When signs of botulism, such as visual problems, appear, the stomach should be pumped out, cathartics should be given, and strychnine and other stimulants should be supplied as needed.

The guilty meal may stay in the stomach for a long time since one of the disease's notable symptoms is the paralysis of the digestive system caused by the toxin ingested (cf. Stiles, loc. cit.). Therefore, even if the patient is not seen for many days after ingesting the hazardous meal, steps should still be taken to empty the stomach.

The Koch Institute in Berlin has created an antitoxic serum.

Although this serum has had positive outcomes in studies on animals, as far as I know, it has never been used in a human epidemic. It is not offered anywhere in this nation.

ADDITIONAL BACTERIAL POISONS

The intriguing scenario presented by Barber demonstrates that there are more avenues for bacterially produced toxins to cause toxic food. Several people had acute gastro-enteritis episodes after consuming milk that contained a deadly toxin made by a white staphylococcus. In practically pure culture, this staphylococcus was found in the udder of the cow that provided the milk. The milk was poisonous when it was used immediately, but only after it had been allowed to stand for many hours at room temperature. The signs and symptoms were those often associated with "ptomain poisoning."

DECOMPOSED AND POISONED FOOD

Every time sensory data suggests that food is more or less disintegrated, there is a widespread perception that it is unwholesome. This viewpoint is reflected in several legal provisions that prohibit the trade of decayed meats, vegetables, and fruits in civilized nations. Unfortunately, there isn't enough data to determine which types or levels of apparent decomposition are the most hazardous. In reality, several foods with great nutritional content, particularly cheeses, are only consumed after undergoing very severe disintegration processes, or "ripening." Just as the disagreeable odors produced by decaying eggs or meat are caused by compounds manufactured by certain species of molds and bacteria, the distinctive smells or fragrances of the different hard and soft cheeses are caused by compounds manufactured by certain species of molds and bacteria. These substances are appropriately considered byproducts of decomposition. In fact, several of the breakdown products produced during the ripening of Brie, Camembert, or Limburger are comparable to, if not the same as, those linked to damaged goods. Again, sour milk is often suggested as a snack or drink for those with fragile health, despite the fact that it contains millions of bacteria and the products of their decomposition. Some of the bacteria that are often involved in milk naturally spoiling have strong ties to pathogenic varieties. It's a common belief that the partial decomposition of meats and game birds is beneficial rather than harmful. Even eggs, a meal whose perceived "freshness" is usually tainted by the early stages of decomposition, are ripened in different ways by the Chinese and consumed as a delicacy after a period of months or years. Pidan, or preserved duck eggs, are kept for months in a paste-like concoction of tea, lime, salt, and wood ashes. They vary significantly from fresh eggs.

The inner membrane of the somewhat darkened shell is covered with a lot of dark green specks. The white is coagulated and dark, much like coffee jelly. The yolk is also coagulated. These eggs have seen an exceptional rise in ammoniacal nitrogen levels, which suggests extensive protein breakdown. The ammoniacal nitrogen content of pidan is much higher than that of the eggs that egg candlers refer to as "black rots."

Therefore, it is clear that bacterial growth in materials used to make food is not always harmful and may, in certain instances, improve the palatability of food without compromising its wholesomeness. It is currently impossible to determine at what stage of the decomposition process a food becomes unfit to use due to the accumulation of poisonous substances within it because little to nothing is known about the correlation of visible signs of decomposition with the presence of poisonous products. There doesn't appear to be a link between a food's inherent dislike and its unwholesomeness. Eggs have a typical nauseating quality under normal circumstances, yet few nitrogenous items have as good a track record for health or have been linked to outbreaks of toxic food as eggs.

On the basis of the facts at hand, it could be tempting to draw the conclusion that dangerous properties are only present in ruined or degraded foods when certain bacteria, such as the previously mentioned B. botulinus, have unintentionally entered them and created precise and specific poisons. However, it would be incorrect to think that all of the byproducts of the common bacteria's breakdown are harmless. It is possible to blame them for no clearly defined acute form of poisoning, but that does not mean that the normal breakdown products do not have any irritating or maybe mildly poisonous effects. Our current understanding of the kind and severity of harm that might result from using damaged food is incomplete and insufficient. Despite this, we are nevertheless required to maintain protective measures that are at least somewhat informed by experience.

CHAPTER NINE

OBSCURE OR UNKNOWN NATURE POISONING

While many and varied causes of toxic food have been covered in the pages that have come before, there are still certain illnesses that are unquestionably related to food but yet have a murky or uncertain etiology.

SICKNESS OR TREMBLES OF MILK

The main symptoms of this illness, which affects both humans and certain higher animals, are severe vomiting and stubborn constipation, which are often accompanied by a subnormal fever. Many situations end in death. In several of the southern and central western states of this nation, it is known to happen relatively rarely at the moment, but during the time of pioneer colonization, it was rather prevalent in areas that are now rarely impacted.

The illness seems to be mostly spread by grazing sheep or cattle with access to certain parcels of land;

these "milksickness" pastures are often widely recognized locally for their hazardous characteristics. Man may get milk sickness by consuming raw milk, butter, or potentially even meat. Although some of the early observers claimed that the illness is self-propagating and may be transferred unrestrictedly from one animal to another, subsequent investigations challenged this theory.

To explain the disease's genesis, several ideas have been put forward. The idea that grazing animals could absorb mineral toxins like arsenic or copper and excrete them in their milk is unsupported by analytical or clinical evidence. There is disagreement about which kinds of plants—many of which are known or believed to be deadly—provide the chemical that gives milk from animals with trembling its lethal nature. In no instance have feeding studies with alleged plants produced outcomes that were clear-cut. While some evidence has been used to support the theory that milk illness is caused by live microorganisms, other evidence contradicts this theory, and the most recent tests in this area did not provide definitive findings. Currently, it is mostly unclear what exactly causes milk sickness.

COMPLEX DISEASES

While not necessarily to be classified as toxic food, diseases caused by the absence rather than the presence of certain food components may nonetheless be addressed here to highlight the intricacy of the food issue. Some observers link at least one illness, pellagra, to the presence of a harmful material or microorganism in the diet, while others attribute it to the lack of certain components required for the healthy preservation of life.

Beriberi. Beriberi is among the most well-documented cases of a disease brought on by an imbalanced or poor diet. This attachment is common among individuals who eat rice cooked in a certain manner as their main or only source of nutrition. According to trade custom, polished white rice has traditionally been regarded as being better than the unpolished kind. The red pericarp, or husk, of the rice grain is removed during the mechanical polishing process, which results in the well-known sickness known as beriberi, which was formerly thought to be an infectious condition. It has been shown that the sickness cannot progress if the husks are added back to the polished grain and consumed as food. Experiments on hens and pigeons reveal that a white rice-only diet results in a condition (polyneuritis of fowls) comparable to beriberi in these species, which may also be stopped or avoided by changing the diet. These findings have led to the conclusion that specific chemicals found in the pericarp of rice grains are necessary for the preservation of health and that their removal from the diet causes nutritional problems. These chemicals go by the moniker "vitamin," although nothing is understood about their chemistry or physiological makeup. Vitamins are probably available in a range of foods in a diverse diet, but if the diet is severely limited, even seemingly insignificant treatment of the food may lead to their eradication. It is unclear how numerous and how different the chemicals are that some authors have categorized as vitamins. There are at least two "determinants"—a fat-soluble and a water-soluble substance—that are considered to be involved in the feeding of growth.

One of the illnesses linked to an imbalanced diet is pellagra, and it has been hypothesized that the recent rise in consumption of highly milled wheat and maize flour devoid of vitamins may be to blame for the disease's recent spread. While some observers agree that a poor diet may increase the risk of developing pellagra, TB, and other illnesses, they do not agree that it is the main contributing factor.

LATHYRISM

A sickness thought to be related to the consumption of chickpeas and pulses has been given the label lathyrism. Although the condition is of a lesser variety than pellagra, nervous symptoms are noticeable and sometimes severe. The sickness is allegedly linked to the exclusive or almost exclusive consumption of legumes and to generally deplorable living circumstances. It is still unknown whether lathyrism is a deficiency illness like beriberi and possibly pellagra, whether it results from consuming specific poisonous legumes mixed with foreign seeds, or whether, in certain circumstances, the legumes themselves may contain poisonous substances produced by unidentified fungus growths.

Favism (from the word "bean") is an acute febrile anemia with jaundice and hemoglobinuria that is exclusive to Italy and has been linked to eating beans or even just smelling the bean plant's flower. There is said to be a clear individual propensity for the disease. No poisonous chemical has been identified in the involved beans, despite the fact that the symptoms are quite severe and seem to indicate acute poisoning. Although it has been hypothesized that either a bacterial infection or a fungal growth on the bean is to blame, neither theory has been backed up by any data.

Scurvy of various types is unquestionably linked to the absence of key essential nutrients in a typical diet. Scurvy may develop aboard ships in the absence of fresh milk, vegetables, fruit juice, and the like. This is a well-known fact. Guinea pigs fed on milk, both raw and cooked, as well as milk plus grain, have shown classic scurvy signs. On the other hand, guinea pigs and rabbits fed a regular diet of green vegetables, hay, and oats were able to develop an experimental type of scurvy after receiving an intravenous injection of certain streptococci. Therefore, some researchers see the proportional contribution of nutrition and infection to the development of human scurvy as being ambiguous.

A medical illness known as rickets or _rachitis_ is somehow linked to a chronic digestive disorder that impairs calcium metabolism. It does not seem likely that rickets is brought on by insufficient calcium in the diet but rather by the bone tissue's inability to utilize the calcium that is sent to it in bodily fluids.

Studies on the disease's origin have not consistently produced consistent findings, and it does not seem viable now to attribute this illness to any specific dietary pattern, such as a diet low in fat or high in carbs or protein. It seems to be true that prolonged consumption of any meal causing a nutritional disruption prevents bone cells from properly absorbing calcium salts.

While there are numerous unanswered questions about the causes of scurvy and rickets, there is little doubt that some dietary deficiency lies at the root of both and that by maintaining proper nutritional circumstances, they may be treated or completely prevented.

THE MOST COMMONLY TOXIC FOODS

In reports of toxic food outbreaks, certain food items appear particularly often. In certain circumstances, the existence of this unique responsibility to do harm is unclear. For instance, vanilla ice cream and vanilla puddings have been linked to so many illnesses that some researchers haven't hesitated to claim that the vanilla itself is hazardous. No solid data exists to support this, however, and a very speculative argument has been put forth that vanilla's reducing effect encourages the development of anaerobic bacteria that generate poisons.

The frequent sourcing of meat from animals carrying parasites hazardous to humans has previously been discussed and is a major factor in the striking regularity with which eating raw meat causes toxic food. In addition to occasionally coming from an infected animal like meat, milk is also a particularly good culture medium for bacteria and can become contaminated during collection or distribution by way of a human carrier. This makes raw milk even more at fault. Foods made with milk, such as ice cream, are often linked to food sickness. It seems likely that bacterial infections rather than metal or flavoring extract poisoning are the main causes of ice cream-related illnesses. These later drugs' accountability is quite troublesome.

The causes of cheese poisoning, which is reportedly extremely common, are rather hazy. It is unclear in the majority of cases whether such poisoning is more frequently caused by initial milk contamination, a pathogenic bacterial invasion of the cheese during preparation, or the formation of toxic substances by bacteria or molds during the ripening process that the cheese goes through.

Unquestionably, sewage pollution of the water where the bivalves are harvested may result in shellfish poisoning from eating oysters, mussels, or clams. In such situations, bacilli of the typhoid or paratyphoid families are often involved. It is debatable whether specific episodes of mussel poisoning that have been documented have been caused by a bacterial infection or whether occasionally healthy or sick mussels acquired from unpolluted water carry a toxin. Similar to this, it is unclear if a certain sea snail (Murex bradatus), which is sometimes used as food, naturally contains a chemical that is dangerous to humans or whether this trait is restricted to infections or the growth of toxigenic bacteria.

Some instances of potato poisoning have been linked to the bacterial proteus bacilli that break down potatoes, while other cases have been linked to the deadly alkaloid solanin, which is allegedly found in large amounts in infected and sprouting potatoes. It's important to remember that many cases of potato poisoning have been linked to eating potato salad that had been mixed up and left out for a while; thus, the risk of contamination with the paratyphoid bacillus or other pathogenic organisms cannot be ruled out. Many investigators are skeptical that solanin has ever really caused potato poisoning.

These examples are adequate to demonstrate that there is a great deal of confusion about the true cause of the problem in a significant number of instances of purported toxic food. Although there has been a shift in thought toward a greater acceptance of the contribution of certain bacteria, particularly those in the paratyphoid group, there is still a significant persistence of unexplained toxic food that requires additional professional examination. One of the goals of this book is to emphasize this necessity and call attention to the many issues that still need to be resolved.

CONCLUSION

Reevaluating our dietary choices and food lifestyle is essential for maintaining a healthy and balanced life. Throughout this exploration of toxic human food, we have learned about the potential dangers associated with certain dietary practices and the negative impacts they can have on our overall well-being.

By understanding the harmful effects of processed foods, high sugar intake, unhealthy fats, and artificial additives, we can make informed decisions about what we consume. It is crucial to prioritize whole, unprocessed foods, such as fruits, vegetables, lean proteins, and whole grains, as they provide essential nutrients and support our body's optimal functioning.

Furthermore, being mindful of portion sizes, practicing moderation, and adopting a balanced approach to eating can significantly contribute to our overall health and well-being. Developing a healthy relationship with food involves listening to our bodies' cues, recognizing hunger and fullness, and nourishing ourselves with nutrient-dense choices.

Remember, this process of reevaluating our dietary choices is a lifelong journey that requires dedication, education, and self-awareness. Consulting with healthcare professionals or nutritionists can provide valuable guidance tailored to individual needs and goals.

By making conscious choices and embracing a sustainable food lifestyle, we can optimize our health, increase our energy levels, and reduce the risk of various chronic diseases. Let us strive to prioritize nourishing our bodies, respecting the food we consume, and cultivating a positive relationship with our dietary choices for a vibrant and fulfilling life.